Y0-BUP-305

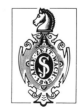

Shen-yi Li En-yu Wang

Endometrial Carcinoma

With the Collaboration of Michihiro Seta

With 67 Figures and 57 Tables

The People's Medical Publishing House Beijing

Springer-Verlag Berlin Heidelberg New York
London Paris Tokyo Hong Kong Barcelona

Authors and Translators

Dr. Shen-yi Li
Associate Professor, Gynecologic Oncology Department
Chief of Medical Affairs Branch

Dr. En-yu Wang
Associate Professor, Gynecologic Oncology Department

Cancer Institute (Hospital)
Chinese Academy of Medical Sciences
Beijing 100021, P.R.China

Original Chinese Edition published by
The People's Medical Publishing House, Beijing, 1988

ISBN 3-540-51273-X Springer-Verlag Berlin Heidelberg New York
ISBN 0-387-51273-X Springer-Verlag New York Berlin Heidelberg

Library of Congress Cataloging-in-Publication Data.
Li, Shen-yi, 1941–
Endometrial carcinoma/Shen-yi Li, En-yu Wang; contributor, Michihiro Seta.
p.cm.
Translation of an original Chinese ed. published by the People's Medical
Pub. House, Beijing, 1988.
Includes bibliographical references.
ISBN 0-387-51273-X (U.S.: alk. paper)
1. Endometrium-Cancer. I. Wang, En-yu, 1942– II. Seta, Michihiro. III. Title.
[DNLM: 1. Uterine Neoplasms.   WP   460   L693e]
RC280.U8L47   1990   616.99′466-dc20   DNLM/DLC   90-9694

Typesetting: Macmillan India Ltd., Bangalore-25, India
2121/3140 (3011)-543210-Printed on acid-free paper.

Dedicated in Gratitude
to Our Teachers

Preface

During the past 20 years, endometrial carcinoma has continued to increase in frequency and it is quite possible that this carcinoma will become the major gynecologic malignancy in the future. For many years, endometrial carcinoma was considered less malignant than other gynecologic malignancies, simple hysterectomy and bilateral salpingo-oophorectomy or surgery combined with radiation being effective in certain circumstances. It is unfortunate to note that the global 5-year survival rate for patients with advanced or recurrent endometrial carcinoma has improved only slightly. Therefore any complacency regarding this 'benign malignancy' should be reconsidered.

There is a growing awareness of the nature of endometrial carcinoma, with advances in our knowledge ranging from its etiology through its epidemiology to its clinical findings. This volume has been designed to fill a hiatus in the literature in China. To achieve this aim, we have attempted to review the world-wide advances on endometrial carcinoma and summarize systematically and comprehensively this common gynecologic malignancy, including the clinical experiences gathered at the Cancer Institute (Hospital) of the Chinese Academy of Medical Sciences since 1958 as well as a brief description of the psychological problems in patients with gynecologic cancers.

We are very grateful to our photographer, Mr. Liu Xi-Chan for the high quality of the photographs. We would also like to express our sincere thanks to the publishers for their care and efficiency in preparing the text and illustrations, and particularly to Dr. Ute Heilmann, who edited the text with much patience and genuine understanding.

Beijing, March 1990   Shen-yi Li
                                                     En-yu Wang

Contents

1 Epidemiology and Etiology

1.1 Epidemiology

Endometrial carcinoma is also called corpus cancer. During the past 20 years there has been a drastic increase in the worldwide incidence of endometrial carcinoma, such that in many areas endometrial carcinoma is now ranked as the second or third most common malignant neoplasm of the female genital tract. The reported incidence varies according to country, area, and race. According to the International Agency for Research on Cancer (1982), incidence rates are especially high in North America and northern Europe and are low in Central America and Asia (Fig. 1.1). The American Cancer Society reported that approximately 37 000 women would develop endometrial carcinoma in 1979. Therefore, this lesion is seen over twice as frequently as carcinoma of the ovary and cervix (Cancer Statistics 1979). Masubuchi et al. (1975) reported 1958 patients with endometrial carcinoma and 38 080 patients with cervical cancer during the 12 years from 1961 to 1972, based on records collected from 33 university hospitals and cancer centers in Japan, giving a ratio of the incidence of endometrial carcinoma to cervical cancer of 1:19.5. In the United States, the ratio of the incidence of endometrial carcinoma to cervical cancer was reported to be 1:2 during the period 1969–1970 (Duun 1974).

Racial differences have been observed such as those between blacks or browns and whites in South Africa, where the ratio of incidence to invasive cervical cancer was 1:8.5 and 2.5:1, respectively. According to the incidence of cancer for the period 1968–1972 in North America, considerable variation exists, the highest being an annual figure of almost 30/100 000 among San Francisco whites. Racial differences such as those between whites and blacks in the San Francisco Bay area, among the inhabitants of New Mexico from European non-Spanish, Spanish and Indian stock, and among inhabitants of the Pacific region – the native Hawaiian, whites, Chinese, Japanese, and Philippines – suggest that the incidence is higher in richer than in poorer communities (Fig 1.2) (Waard and Oettle 1965; Waard 1982). It is interesting that the incidence in groups of similar ethnic origin living in different countries is very variable; for example, the incidence among the Japanese in Hawaii is much higher than those in Japan (Fig. 1.3) (IARC 1982).

In recent years a true epidemic of endometrial carcinoma has occurred in several parts of the United States (Weiss et al. 1976). This is firmly documented for the San Francisco Bay area, where the annual incidence for the 50- to 74-year age group tripled in 15 years (Austin and Roe 1979). Something similar is true for

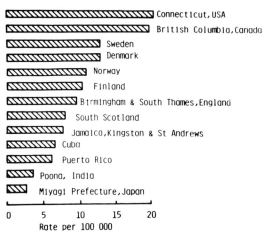

Fig. 1.1. Age-adjusted incidence of endometrial carcinoma in selected countries (IARC 1982)

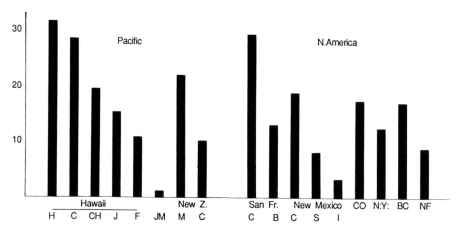

Fig. 1.2. Standardized incidence rates of endometrial carcinoma in some populations of the Pacific region and North America.

Hawaii: *H*, Hawaiian; *C*, Caucasian; *CH*, Chinese; *J*, Japanese; *F*, Filipino origin; *JM*, Japan Miyagi prefecture; **New Zealand**: *M*, Maoris; *C*, non-Maoris (mainly Caucasian); **San Francisco Bay area**: *C*, non-Spanish Caucasians; *S*, Spanish origin; *I*, Indian. *CO*, Conneticut; *NY*, upstate New York; *BC*, British Columbia; *NF*, New Foundland. (Waard 1982)

South Africa. In 1965, Waard and Oettle reported that the number of endometrial carcinoma cases at the large Baragwanath Hospital near Johannesburg seemed to be on the increase. They predicted a further rise due to the improving socioeconomic circumstances of the urban blacks, and further statistics lead to the conclusion that this prediction was probably correct (Table 1.1).

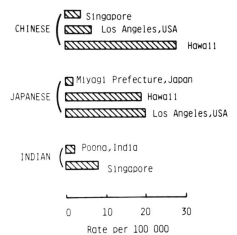

Fig. 1.3. Age-adjusted incidence of endo-metrial carcinoma in Chinese, Japanese, and Indians living in various countries (IARC 1982)

Table 1.1. Endometrial cancer diagnosed in Baragwanath Hospital, which serves the black population of Soweto near Johannesburg. (Adapted from Waard 1982)

Period	Number of cases
1951–1956 (6 years)	0
1957–1962 (6 years)	12
1968–1973 (6 years)	41
1974–1978 (5 years)	76

It has been found that the incidence ratio for endometrial carcinoma to cancer of the cervix is very different in various countries, areas, and races. The incidence of endometrial carcinoma is much higher than that of cancer of the cervix in Alameda, Connecticut, in whites in the Bay area, United States, in Israel, and in Malta. The incidence of endometrial carcinoma is lower and an opposite ratio even appears in Colombia, India, Cuba, and Japan (Table 1.2).

The analysis of cancer registry from Huaxi Medical University and Cancer Institute Hospital, Chinese Academy of Medical Sciences, Beijing, China, also shows that the incidence of endometrial carcinoma has tended to increase (Table 1.3) (Li 1988).

From the above it would appear that either the increased incidence of this disease or increased number of cases in some hospitals could be recognized, and the change in ratio of cases of endometrial carcinoma and cervical cancer could implicate an increase of endometrial carcinoma. Of course, there are several important factors which cannot be excluded in analyzing the increased incidence

Table 1.2. Incidence per 100 000 of endometrial carcinoma and cervical cancer

Geographic area	Cervical cancer	Endometrial carcinoma
United States		
Alameda	12.3	33.3
Bay area	12.1	29.3
Conneticut	9.8	17.8
Israel	4.5	10.8
Malta	7.1	13.1
Brazil, Sao Paulo	27.5	8.5
Colombia, Cali	62.8	5.1
Cuba	19.5	10.9
India	23.2	1.3
Nigeria. Ibadan	21.6	1.6
Japan	13.8	1.3
Osaka	16.2	0.9
Norway	18.1	9.7
Poland, Warsaw	21.5	9.5
United Kingdom,		
Birmingham	12.6	8.5

Table 1.3. Incidence ratio of endometrial carcinoma to cervical cancer in China

	Period	Ratio
Hua Xi Medical	1955–1966	1 : 18.1
University	1967–1978	1 : 6
Cancer Institute	1958–1969	1 : 44
Hospital	1970–1981	1 : 18.5

of endometrial carcinoma. Greenblatt and Stoddard (1978) suggested several reasons for the increase in incidence:

1. Greater availability of medical care: more women are provided with medical care; therefore more cancers are detected.
2. More women reach the critical age for the development of endometrial carcinoma.
3. A broadening of criteria for the diagnosis of endometrial carcinoma by the inclusion of severe dysplasia, a typical adenomatous hyperplasia, carcinoma in situ, and the so-called well-differentiated endometrial carcinoma in the cancer registry as adenocarcinoma.

4. A worldwide increase in endometrial carcinoma due possibly to environmental and unknown factors.

   However, it is clear that despite these factors there has been a trend toward
increased incidence of endometrial carcinoma.

1.2 Etiology

Etiologic investigation into endometrial carcinoma has been vigorously pursued
in the past 30 years. Studies on the relationship between steroids and endometrial carcinoma have made great progress, but the cause of disease remains
unclear. However, some risk factors associated with endometrial carcinoma have
been noted. These include age, obesity, nulliparity, late menopause, hypertension, diabetes mellitus, ovarian estrogen-producing tumors, ovarian dysgenesis,
polycystic ovarian syndrome, oral contraceptives, and exogenous estrogen. The
majority of these factors may cause excessive estrogen production, and prolonged unopposed estrogen stimulation of the endometrium appears causally
related to the development of endometrial carcinoma.

1.2.1 Age

Generally, endometrial carcinoma occurs in the postmenopausal period, primarily in the age group of 55–59 years. The age range is from the 2nd to the 9th
decade. Only 20%–25% of the patients with endometrial carcinoma are premenopausal, 2%–5% of whom are under the age of 40 years. The incidence
obviously declines over the age of 70 years (Mattingly 1977). A 1958–1981
Cancer Institute Hospital, Beijing, study of 449 women with endometrial
carcinoma found that the age range extends from 29 to 76 years, with 45%
(202/449 cases) of the patients in the age group of 50–59 years, 34.7% of patients
(156/449 cases) premenopausal, and 10.2% of patients (45/449 cases) under the
age of 40 years (L 1988).

1.2.2 Obesity

Obesity is associated with an increased risk in some patients with endometrial
carcinoma. Damon (1960) demonstrated a 13% increase in the mean body
weight of patients with endometrial carcinoma compared with control patients
of similar height. Wynder et al. (1966) reported that women overweight by
21–50 lb have a threefold greater risk of developing endometrial carcinoma and
women overweight by over 50 lb have a tenfold greater risk of developing
endometrial carcinoma. Similar studies in Boston demonstrated 1.8 times the
risk for women in the upper third of the weight distribution, increasing to 2.4

Table 1.4. Weight of women with endometrial carcinoma and of control subjects aged 50–59 years. (Modified from Wynder et al. 1966)

Weight	% women with endometrial cancer ($n=90$)	% control women ($n=150$)	Relative risk, cases: controls
Below average weight by			
21 lb or more	7	12	0.9
10–20 lb	9	20	0.7
3–9 lb	10	19	0.9
Average weight ± 2 lb	8	13	1.0
Above average weight by			
3–9 lb	9	9	1.6
10–20 lb	11	9	2.0
21–50 lb	28	15	3.1
51 lb or more	18	3	9.8

times the risk for patients in the top 15% of the weight distribution (MacMahon 1974).

In addition, 32.6% of patients were obese in a group of endometrial carcinoma patients in the Cancer Institute Hospital, Beijing. Wynder et al. (1966) summarized the distribution of body weight in a group of patients with endometrial carcinoma and matched controls (Table 1.4).

1.2.3 Nulliparity

Nulliparity is commonly associated with an increased risk of developing endometrial carcinoma. Some papers have reported that 24%–31% of patients with endometrial carcinoma were nulliparous. Nulliparity was associated with twice the risk of development of endometrial carcinoma compared with primipara and three times the risk of women with five children (Masubichi and Nemoto 1972; MacMahon 1974). Lang et al. (1978) reported that 68.5% (74/108 cases) of patients with endometrial carcinoma in Beijing Union Hospital were women with primary and secondary infertility. Li (1988) also reported 25% of patients with endometrial carcinoma having primary infertility. Some authors comment that pregnancy is a powerful factor in protecting against endometrial carcinoma, which is perhaps related to the shedding of the endometrium which occurs at parturition, protecting the endometrium from estrogen stimulation for one or several years. The more pregnancies a woman has, the greater is her protection from endometrial carcinoma. However, this protection must be absent in women with infertility.

1.2.4 Late Menopause

Late menopause has been recognized as a risk factor in the development of endometrial carcinoma. Menopause after the age of 52 years has a 2.4 times greater risk for the development of endometrial carcinoma compared with menopause before the age of 49 years (Elwood et al. 1977). Screening 5966 women in the Beijing area of China showed that 938 women were postmenopausal, the median age of menopause was 47.8 years and 46.7 years for urban women and rural women respectively, and that menopause occurred at 50 years of age in 25.7% (Wu 1982). Statistical studies of 418 patients with endometrial carcinoma in the Cancer Institute Hospital demonstrated that 296 patients were menopausal, the median age of menopause was 49.3 years, and the menopause in 56% of them occurred at over 50 years of age (Li et al. 1988).

Therefore, it is generally accepted that spontaneous menopause is later in patients with endometrial carcinoma than in normal matched controls, so long-term estrogen stimulation to the endometrium occurred.

1.2.5 Diabetes Mellitus, Hypertension, and Associated Internal Medical Diseases

Diabetes mellitus and hypertension are frequently associated with endometrial carcinoma. Diabetes or a diabetic tendency is present in 11%–45% of patients with endometrial carcinoma and the incidence of hypertension varies from 25% to 60% (Van Nagell et al. 1972). Women with a history of diabetes had a 2.8-fold risk compared with the controls (Elwood et al. 1977). Frick et al. (1973) reported 5.3%–41% of patients with endometrial carcinoma had abnormal carbohydrate intolerance and 25% of the patients will have hypertension or arteriosclerotic heart disease. Fox and Sen (1970), comparing patients with endometrial carcinoma with matched controls, found a statistically significant higher incidence of hypertension in patients with endometrial carcinoma than in the controls, but only at the $P = 0.05$ level. Hypertension is prevalent in the elderly, obese woman and does not appear to be a significant risk factor by itself. A combination of obesity, hypertension, and diabetes mellitus, called a trilogy of endometrial carcinoma, commonly appears in some patients. The pituitary functional disorder may be a common cause of endometrial carcinoma and metabolic abnormality, but is not generally accepted due to lack of sufficient experimental evidence.

In addition, there is a slightly higher frequency of arthritis and hypothyroidism in patients with endometrial carcinoma compared with controls (Elwood et al. 1977). Husslein et al. (1978) reported that one patient with endometrial carcinoma was diagnosed 20 months after successful renal transplantation. Immunosuppressive states and immunodeficiency diseases are highly correlated with the development of malignancy.

1.2.6 Ovarian Tumors and Ovarian Diseases

Endometrial carcinoma may develop in patients with ovarian hormone-secreting tumors. Gusberg and Kardon (1971), Mansell and Hertig (1955), Norris and Taylor (1968), and Greene (1957) reported that 9%–27% of patients with ovarian granulosa theca cell tumor would associate with endometrial carcinoma since it was first described by Novak and Yui in 1936. Gusberg and Kardon reported that, of 115 patients with so-called ovarian-feminizing tumors, 21% were found to have endometrial carcinoma and 43% had complications of precancerous changes and carcinoma in situ. It is well known that granulosa theca cell tumor may produce high-level circulating estrogen unopposed by progesterone, and estrogen may stimulate the endometrium continuously (McDonald et al. 1977a).

It has been known for many years that endometrial carcinoma may occur in patients with polycystic ovary syndrome (Stein-Leventhal syndrome) and ovarian dysgenesis (Turner's syndrome). Endometrial carcinoma has been reported to be as high as 25% in patients with Stein-Leventhal syndrome. Chronic anovulation associated with unopposed estrogen stimulation to the endometrium increases the risk of endometrial carcinoma in these patients.

Until 1978, 14 patients with endometrial carcinoma associated with Turner's syndrome had been reported (McCarty et al. 1978; Ostor et al. 1978). It is generally accepted that the long-term supplemental estrogen that is given to these patients in childhood can increase the risk of endometrial carcinoma. McDonald et al. (1977a) reported that induction of ovulation with wedge resection of the ovaries and administration of clomiphene citrate will reverse the overstimulation of the endometrium.

1.2.7 Oral Contraceptives

Silverberg and Makowski (1975) stated that an increased incidence of endometrial carcinoma in young women became evident in users of sequential oral contraceptives. Endometrial carcinoma occurred especially in those products with a combination of very potent estrogen and weak progestogen, as progestogen does not possess the necessary protective properties. These tumors when associated with contraceptives are characterized by low grade and stage, rare myometrial invasion, and good prognosis. It is of interest to learn that conjugated oral contraceptives can decrease the incidence of endometrial carcinoma. Weiss and Sayvetz (1980) studied 117 patients with endometrial carcinoma aged 35–54 years. These patients were compared with 395 controls. The risk ratio increased to 7 after sequential contraceptives were taken, but conjugated oral contraceptives may decrease the risk ratio to 0.5.

1.2.8 Exogenous Estrogen

Long-term unopposed estrogen supplementation may increase the risk of endometrial carcinoma, and the longer duration and the higher dosage, the higher the increase in risk. The risk ratio of the development of endometrial carcinoma with exogenous estrogen ranges from 2.0 to 13.9 (Mack et al. 1976; Gray et al. 1977). Ziel and Finkle (1975) took the lead in making more thorough retrospective and prospective investigations into this issue. They evaluated the risk factor of estrogen in patients with endometrial carcinoma at the Kaiser Foundation Health Plan in Los Angeles. The carcinoma cases were compared with 186 controls who had intact uteri, and a risk ratio of 7.6 was noted. About 57% of the patients with endometrial carcinoma had taken estrogen as against 15% of controls. If the conjugated estrogen was taken for 1–4.9 years, the risk ratio was 5.6, which will increase to 13.9 if estrogen is taken for more than 7 years.

Mack et al. (1976) reported their evaluation of relationship between estrogen and endometrial carcinoma in a retirement community. There were 63 patients with endometrial carcinoma and 252 controls in the same community. They found that 81% of patients had taken estrogen compared with 42% of controls. The risk ratio for those taking estrogen was 8.0 and for those taking conjugated estrogen 5.6.

There have been more articles evaluating the use of exogenous estrogen in patients with endometrial carcinoma. Gray et al. (1977) surveyed 205 patients with endometrial carcinoma from 1947 to 1976 and compared them with 205 controls who had had hysterectomy for benign diseases. They found that 26% of the patients had taken estrogen compared with 15% of the controls. The risk ratio for conjugated estrogen was 3.1, but for all others it was 2.1. The risk ratio increased with years use of the drug; the difference was only signigicant after 10 years, however. Many criticisms have been directed at these studies including the inappropriate choice of controls. Horwitz and Feinstein (1978) questioned studies that have shown a large risk ratio between endometrial carcinoma and exogenous estrogen. They noted a bias in selecting controls. They evaluated their patients by using two groups of controls. With conventional controls, similar to in other studies, 29% of the patients with endometrial carcinoma had taken estrogen compared with 3% of the controls, the ratio being 11.98. When more appropriate alternative controls and when patients who had had curettage or hysterectomy were used to overcome bias, the ratio was reduced to 1.7.

The issue of cause-effect relationship between estrogen and endometrial carcinoma remains unsettled because of the varying statistical methods and variable results. (McDonald 1976)

1.2.9 Previous Pelvic Irradiation

Previous pelvic irradiation may lead to a higher incidence of endometrial carcinoma. It is possible that the "underlying factors" for which they were irradiated may be irritated to cause endometrial carcinoma (MacMahon 1974). There is another opinion in the literature evaluating the relationship between previous irradiation and endometrial carcinoma. Rodriquez and Hart (1982) stated that previous radiotherapy should not be a carcinogenic factor as the endometrium had been destroyed by irradiation.

Of the 449 patients with endometrial carcinoma in the Cancer Hospital, Beijing, 2.2% (10 cases) were found to have previous irradiation history for the treatment of cervical cancer (Li et al. 1988).

Like other types of neoplasm, the etiology of endometrial carcinoma is still unsolved. In recent years, there has been considerable emphasis on the role of environmental and host factors in the causation of human cancer. At the symposium of Host Factors in Human Carcinogenesis held by IARC in 1981, Weinstein pointed out that specific environmental and host factors such as genetic factors, carcinogens, hormones, viruses, nutrition, and some inhibitors can play either an enhancing or an inhibiting role in the carcinogenic process (Weinstein 1982). Armstrong (1982) suggested that endogenous hormones probably do not initiate cancer directly but may influence carcinogenesis by facilitation or inhibition of endogenous production of carcinogens; affect the metabolic activation or inactivation of carcinogens; alter the susceptibility of tissues to the initiation of cancer; promote the development of clinical cancer from initiated cells; and alter the body's capacity to eliminate initiated cells. Evidence exists for a role of endogenous hormones in cancers of the salivary gland, colon and rectum, liver, gallbladder, pancreas, breast, cervix uteri, corpus uteri, ovary, prostate, testis, kidney, thyroid and pituitary glands, and malignant melanoma.

Studies on the relationship between steroids and certain types of hormone-dependent tumors, especially those of the breast and endometrium, have made much progress. Based on the aforementioned high-risk factors, it is suggested that the development of endometrial carcinoma is associated with long-term, unopposed estrogen stimulation. Therefore, it is important to take into account the circulating "hormone environment" and factors that may modify it.

1.2.10 Summary

Analysis of the high-risk factors described above indicates that this disease is related to a long-term and constant irritation of the unopposed estrogen to the endometrium. The following sections review the literature on this subject.

1.2.10.1 Source of Circulating Estrogens

1.2.10.1.1 Normal Young Women

In normal young women, the circulating estrogen is provided by theca cells and corpus luteum cells in the ovary. The most important estrogens, including estradiol (E_2), estrone (E_1), and estriol (E_3), are secreted by the ovary. Their relative potencies of $E_2 : E_1 : E_3$ are approximately $100 : 10 : 3$. These hormones are synthesized from acetate or cholesterol by way of progesterone and testosterone or androstenedione. Testosterone is converted to β-estradiol by several optional pathways. One involves the oxidation of C-19 to yield 17-hydroxytestosterone followed by the complete removal of the $-CH_3$ at C-10 and aromatization of the A-ring. This step leads to the formation of estrone, which is reversibly convertible to estradiol. Some of the circulating E_2 is provided by the peripheral transformation of testosterone by a process of aromatization. Only a small amount is probably secreted by the adrenal cortex. E_1 is also recognized to be of ovarian origin and E_1 in a lesser amount originates in the extraglandular oxidation of E_2 since the estrogen is metabolized principally via E_1.

The amount of E_1 produced by peripheral aromatization of Δ^4-androstene-3,17-dione (Adione) may provide as much as 50% of the daily production (Siiteri and MacDonald 1973). The synthesis pathway of estrogen is shown in Fig. 1.4 (Fishman et al. 1960; Gurpide et al. 1962).

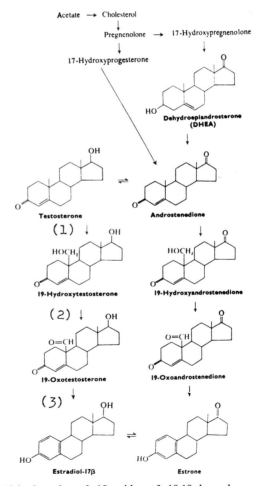

Fig. 1.4. Biogenesis of estrogens. *1*, 19-hydroxylase; *2*, 19-oxidase; *3*, 10,19-desmolase

1.2.10.1.2 Postmenopausal Women

In postmenopausal women, the ovary discontinues its estrogen production almost totally, but it may continue to produce androgens. Two possibilities may be considered concerning the extraglandular production of E_2: either the aromatization of testosterone or the reduction of E_1. E_1 is derived from the peripheral formation of plasma Adione and most of the circulating Adione is synthesized at the adrenal cortex. It seems that the source of estrogen in postmenopausal women is different from that in premenopausal women. The levels of circulating E_2 and E_1 are in general lower than those observed at the follicular phase of the normal menstrual cycle in young women. The levels of E_1 surpass those of E_2 in the approximate proportion of $2:1$ or $3:1$. In the follicular phase of young women, the levels of E_2 are equal to or greater than those of E_1, the concentration of E_1 and the relationship between E_1 and Adione in normal postmenopausal women being similar to values found in castrated women (Barlow et al. 1969; Longcope 1971; Saez et al. 1972; Judd et al. 1974; Greenblatt et al. 1976; Vermeulen 1976; Samoljik et al. 1977; Vermeulen and Verdonck 1978).

Siiteri and MacDonald (1973) investigated the production rate of E_1 derived from Adione and the total E_1 production rate, and they demonstrated that both values are practically identical, i.e. 45.4 vs. 46.3 $\mu g/24$ h, respectively.

It may be concluded that the major source of estrogen in postmenopausal women is the peripheral formation of E_1 from plasma Adione and not from ovarian or adrenal secretion. James et al. (1978) have demonstrated that the injection of physiologic doses of Adione into postmenopausal women produces a rapid and manifest increase in circulating E_1 and sometimes also in E_2.

It is generally accepted that, in postmenopause, E_1 peripherally produced through aromatization of Adione seems to be the main source of estrogen, and the synthesis of E_2 from aromatization of testosterone or the reduction of E_1 must be comparatively very small.

Although estrone sulfate (E_1S) is the principal estrogen in the blood of men and menopausal women, only very little is known about the biologic role of E_1S and estradiol sulfate (E_2S). Recently it has been demonstrated that E_1S is also the most abundant plasma estrogen at menopause. Most E_1S and E_2S are peripherally synthesized from nonconjugated E_1 and E_2. The liver appears to be the most active organ for sulfation. In some target organs of estrogens, like the human endometrium, activity of sulfotransferase has also been demonstrated, showing a significant increase during the secretory phase. Nevertheless, E_1S must not be considered exclusively a metabolite of excretion, since it has been demonstrated that in endometrium and in certain areas of the CNS the E_1S is easily hydrolyzed to E_1 and E_2. It has also been demonstrated that in plasma E_1S circulates bound to proteins, suggesting that E_1S might be considered an inactive plasma reservoir of potentially active estrogens (Boström and Wengle 1967; Brown and Smyth 1971; Loriaux et al. 1971; Rosenthal et al. 1972; Ruder et al. 1972; Payne et al. 1973; Hawkins and Oakey 1974; Buirchell and Hähnel 1975;

Hobkirk et al. 1975; Gurpide et al. 1976; CaristrÃ¶m and skÃ¶ldefors 1977; Nunez et al. 1977; Wright et al. 1978; Pack et al. 1979; Roberts et al. 1980).

1.2.10.2 Tissue Responsible for Peripheral Aromatization and the Regulatory Mechanism of Peripheral Aromatization

Peripheral aromatization should include the following biologic pathways:

1. Peripheral biosynthesis takes place with certain reversible oxidoreduction processes between Adione and testosterone and between E_1 and E_2. The reduced compounds (testosterone and E_2) are biologically much more active than the corresponding oxidated steroids (Adione and E_1).
2. Another extraglandular conversion is an irreversible process responsible for the change in the type of activity of the steroid by transformation of an androgen (T_1, Adione) into the corresponding estrogens (E_2 and E_1). Experiments performed both in vitro and in vivo suggest that adipose tissue may be the tissue responsible for extraglandular aromatization of androgen in humans (Grodin et al. 1973; Siiteri and MacDonald 1973; Nimrod and Ryan 1975; Riskallah et al. 1975; Longcope et al. 1976; Longcope et al. 1978; Perel and Killinger 1979; Forney et al. 1981).

Perel and Killinger (1979) have demonstrated that aromatase is present in adipocytes and in fibrovascular stroma of human adipose tissue. Vermeulen and Verdonck (1978) have found that levels of E_1 and E_2 correlate positively with the degree of obesity in postmenopausal women. Ackerman et al. (1981) have demonstrated that in vitro the cells of the fibrovascular stroma of adipose tissue are capable of converting Adione into E_1 and also E_1 into E_2, this latter change occurring after 48 h of incubation. From this experiment it may be deduced that human adipose tissue contains aromatase and 17β-reductase.

Siiteri and MacDonald (1973) reported that postmenopausal women with obesity and vaginal bleeding of uterine origin have a transfer constant from Adione to E_1 approximately twice that obtained from similar studies performed on the normal postmenopausal group.

Recent studies demonstrate that nonsignificant statistical differences exist between both the plasma levels of E_1 and E_2 and the conversion factor of Adione into E_1 in postmenopausal women with endometrial carcinoma, when these patients as well as their respective normal controls are carefully matched according to total body weight. In other words, the increase in circulating E_1 and E_2 levels and in the conversion factor of Adione to E_1 in women with endometrial carcinoma is mainly due to obesity and not to the presence of tumor (MacDonald et al. 1978; Judd et al. 1980; Davidson et al. 1981). It has been demonstrated that obesity may be the important factor in conversion of Adione to E_1.

Schindler et al. (1972) followed by Forney et al. (1981) discovered that the ability to produce E_1 per gram of adipose tissue in women with hyperplasia or endometrial carcinoma is significantly greater than that in control women of comparable weight. It may be that certain metabolic hormones like insulin, corticoids, and prolactin take part in this regulation of peripheral aromatization of estrone.

It is concluded that all abnormal conditions presenting an increased peripheral aromatization of androgen like obesity or certain metabolic hormones may be considered risk factors for the development of endometrial carcinoma.

1.2.10.3 Sex Hormone Binding Globulin and Transport of Sex Steroids

Mercier et al. (1965) announced the identification of a protein in human plasma behaving electrophoretically like a β-globulin. Sex hormone binding globulin (SHBG) was later assigned to this protein. This protein binds with different affinities, the 17β-hydroxylated sex steroids like T, E_2, 5α-dihydrotestosterone (DHT), and some androstene and androstanediols. Circulating steroids bind to SHBG and also show a high degree of binding to plasma albumin. The binding mechanism with albumin seems to be different from that of SHBG, since it has great capacity but very low affinity. In normal conditions, the free fraction of steroids is estimated as being only 1%–3% of the total and can diffuse freely to the target tissues, thus performing their biologic activities. The bio-availability of plasma E_2 and testosterone would depend on their concentration and on the binding capacity of circulating SHBG (Burke and Anderson 1972; Hammond et al. 1980; Pardridge et al. 1980).

Raynaud et al. (1971) suggested the existence of a high-affinity and low-capacity estrogen-binding protein (E_2BP). The existence of E_2BP has also been supported by Tisman and Wu SJG (1976), Algard et al. (1978), and O'Brien et al. (1982). It is differentiated from SHBG by its isoelectric elution pH, its sedimentation value, and its steroid specificity. It has a high affinity for E_2, diethylstilbestrol, and, to a lesser extent, for E_1. DHT and testosterone, which have high affinities for SHBG, show no affinity for E_2BP. The implications of E_2BP in normal and pathologic states remain to be determined.

The plasma concentration of SHBG is markedly different between the sexes, being about twice as great in women as in men. In prepubertal children of either sex, SHBG levels are higher than those of adult men and similar to those found in normal adult women. SHBG falls significantly at puberty in boys while the values are maintained or rise slightly in girls. After menopause, SHBG diminishes to values comparable to those of normal adult men (Vermeulen et al. 1969; Rosenfield 1971; Duignan 1976; Dennis et al. 1977; Egloff et al. 1981).

Administration of estrogens (natural or synthetic), antiestrogens, and thyroid hormones increases the levels of SHBG, while androgens and somatotropins diminish them (Bird et al. 1969; Vermeulen et al. 1969; Ruder et al. 1971; Westphal 1971; De moor et al. 1972; Rosner 1972; Kley et al. 1973; Dennis et al. 1977; Sakai et al. 1978; Fex et al. 1981). A drop in SHBG levels has been correlated with degree of obesity in postmenopausal women (O'Dea et al. 1979;

Nisker et al. 1980; Davidson et al. 1981). Davidson et al. (1981), studying 25 postmenopausal women with endometrial carcinoma and matching the results with those obtained in healthy women of similar age and body weight, have demonstrated a positive correlation between the degree of obesity and levels of "total" and "free" E_2 in both groups and a negative correlation with respect to values of circulating SHBG. Postmenopausal and obese women, since in this case an increase in circulating estrogens is observed, do not show a subsequent corresponding increase in SHBG, the mechanisms of which are as yet unknown. It may be concluded that obesity in postmenopausal women implies a double risk for endometrial carcinoma, since it produces a rise in circulating estrogens through an increase in peripheral aromatization and a rise in "free" E_2 due to the decrease in plasma SHBG. It may, therefore, be stated that the increase in estrogen produced by obesity at menopause tends toward the development of endometrial carcinoma in this high-risk group.

1.2.10.4 Synergism of Estrogen and Progesterone to Endometrium

The large decrease in progesterone may cause unopposed estrogen stimulation of the endometrium, thus increasing the risk of endometrial carcinoma, even its absence in postmenopausal women, especially those with obesity or functional abnormality in the ovary. It is well known that the histologic changes in the endometrium in the normal menstrual cycle are induced by the ovarian hormones from day to day during a normal cycle. In brief, estrogen stimulates the proliferation of endometrium manifested by the growth and proliferation of the glands and stromal cells. Progestogen can greatly increase the proliferative endometrium. The glands continue to grow, become increasingly corkscrew-shaped, and secrete.

Based on experimental data, it is indicated that progestins counteract some of the estrogen activity. For instance, E_2 promotes cellular proliferation, while progesterone opposes it. Tseng and Gurpide (1975a, b), Gurpide (1978a, b), and Gurpide and Marks (1981) demonstrated in perfusion experiments with human endometrium that progesterone and certain synthetic progestins, like medroxyprogesterone acetate, decrease the levels of E_2 receptors (E_2R) and increase the activity of 17β-hydroxysteroid dehydrogenase, which is responsible for the conversion of E_2 into E_1. Both progestational effects decrease the specific activity of E_2R at the cellular level, making the access of E_2 to the nucleus difficult, whereas both intracellular conversion of E_2 into E_1 and the diffusion of the latter, as E_1 or E_1S, toward the extracellular compartment are facilitated. Tseng and Liu (1981) have demonstrated in vitro that progesterone and medroxyprogesterone acetate increase the activity of sulfotransferase in the human endometrium, thus favoring the conversion of E_1 and E_2 into E_1S and E_2S. In other words, through their effect on sulfotransferase and 17β-dehydrogenase, the progestins play an intracellular antiestrogenic role, protecting the endometrium from excessive stimulation by circulating E_2.

As mentioned above, the mechanism of developing endometrial carcinoma by steroid hormones may be deduced as follows:

In postmenopausal women with the resultant increased risk of developing endometrial carcinoma, the rise in circulating estrogen through an increase in peripheral processes of aromatization, especially the transformation of Adione into E_1 and due to the decrease in plasma SHBG, would stimulate the endometrium continuously and result in endometrial hyperplasia.

At present, there is no direct evidence that estrogens are carcinogenic in humans. The exact mechanisms of developing endometrial carcinoma caused by estrogen are still under investigation. The estrogen source, mechanism of effect on the estrogen levels, endometrial hyperplasia, and developing endometrial carcinoma are shown in Fig. 1.5

Premenopausal women including those under 40 years of age, obesity, nulliparity, diabetes mellitus, and hypertension are also believed to be higher risk factors for the development of endometrial carcinoma. Of the 37 young women with endometrial carcinoma examined by Crissman et al. (1981), 37.7% were obese, 37.5% were nulliparous, 25% had hypertension, and 81% had a history of abnormal vaginal bleeding. Of the 34 women with endometrial carcinoma under 40 years of age reviewed from 1958 to 1981 in the Cancer Institute Hospital, of Beijing, 78% were nulliparous and 91% had abnormal vaginal bleeding (Li 1988).

Endometrial carcinomas rarely occur in ovulating premenopausal women. There are, however, certain conditions in premenopausal women that could lead to chronic anovulation with an increased risk of endometrial carcinoma. Polycystic ovarian syndrome predisposes young girls to endometrial carcinoma. Jackson and Dockerty (1957) reported that 37% of their 42 patients with polycystic ovarian syndrome developed endometrial carcinoma. Notably all but 4 of the 51 cases of endometrial carcinoma associated with polycystic ovarian

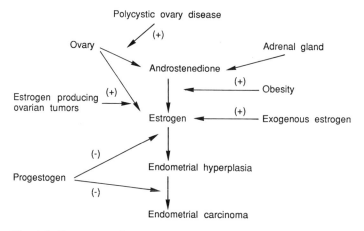

Fig. 1.5. Estrogen and endometrial carcinoma

syndrome reported by Feckner and Kaufman (1974) were well-differentiated adenocarcinomas. Most importantly, none had metastasis beyond the uterus (Feckner and Kaufman 1974; MacDonald et al. 1978).

References

Ackerman GE, Smith ME, Mendelson CR et al. (1981) Aromatization of androstenedione by human adipose tissue stromal cells in monolayer culture. J Clin Endocrinol Metab 53:412–417

Algard FT, Montessori GA, Van Netten JP, Munn M (1978) Is there a high-affinity estrogen binder in human serum? Clin Chem 24:1848–1849

Armstrong B (1982) Endocrine factors in human carcinogenesis. In: Bartsch H, Armstrong B (eds) Host factors in human carcinogenesis. IARC Lyon, p 193–221

Austin DE, Roe KM (1979) Increase in cancer of the corpus uteri in the San Francisco-Oakland standard metropolitan statistical area, 1960–1975. JNCI 62:13–16

Barlow JJ, Emerson K, Saxena BN (1969) Estradiol production after ovariectomy of carcinoma of the breast. Relevance to the treatment of menopausal women. N Engl J Med 280:633–637

Bird Ch E, Green RN, Clark AF (1969) Effect of the administration of estrogen on the disappearance of ^{3}H-testosterone in the plasma of human subjects. J Clin Endocrinol Metab 29:123–126

Boström H, Wengle B (1967) Studies on ester sulfates 23. Distribution of phenol and steroid sulphokinase in adult human tissues. Acta Endocrinol 56:691–704

Brown JB, Smyth BJ (1971) Oestrone sulfate – the major circulating oestrogen in the normal menstrual cycle. J Reprod Fertil 24:142

Buirchell BJ, Hähnell R (1975) Metabolism of estradiol-17β in human endometrium during the menstrual cycle. J Steroid Biochem 6:1489

Burke CW, Anderson DC (1972) Sex-hormone-binding-globulin is an oestrogen amplifier. Nature 240:38–40

Cancer Statistics (1979) CA Cancer J Clin 29:6

Cariström K, Sköldefors H (1977) Determination of total oestrone in peripheral serum from nonpregnant humans. J Steroid Biochem 8:1127–1128

Crissman JD, Azoury RS, Barnes AE, Schelhas HF (1981) Endometrial cancer in women 40 years of age or younger. Obstet Gynecol 57:699–704

Damon A (1960) Host factors in cancer of the breast and uterine cervix and corpus. JNCI 24:483–516

Davidson BJ, Gambone JC, LaGasse LD et al. (1981) Free estradiol in postmenopausal women with and without endometrial cancer. J Clin Endocrinol Metab 52:404–408

De Moor P, Hayns W, Bouillion R (1972) Growth hormone and the steroid binding β-globulin of human plasma. J Steroid Biochem 3:593–600

Dennis M, Horst HJ, Krieg M, Voigt KD (1977) Plasma sex hormone-binding globulin binding capacity in benign prostatic hypertrophy and prostatic carcinoma: comparison with an age dependent rise in normal human males. Acta Endocrinol 84:207–214

Duignan NM (1976) Polycystic ovarian disease. Br J Obstet Gynaecol 83:593–602

Duun J (1974) Geographic consideration of endometrial cancer. Gynecol Oncol 2:114–121

Egloff M, Vranckx R, Tardivel-Lacombe J, Degrelle H (1981) Immunochemical characterization and quantitation of human sex steroid binding plasma protein. Steroids
37:455–462

Elwood JM, Cole P, Rothman KJ, Kaplan SD (1977) Epidemiology of endometrial
cancer. JNCI 59:1055–1060

Feckner RF, Kaufman RH (1974) Endometrial adenocarcinoma in Stein-Leventhal
syndrome. Cancer 34:444–452

Fex G, Adielsson G, Mattson W (1981) Oestrogen-like effects of tamoxifen on the
concentration of proteins in plasma. Acta Endocrinol 97:109–113

Fishman J, Bradlow HL, Gallagher RF (1960) Oxidative metabolism of estradiol. J Biol
Chem 235:3104

Forney JP, Milewich L, Chen GT et al. (1981) Aromatization of androstenedione to
estrone by human adipose tissue in vitro. Correlation with adipose tissue mass, age,
and endometrial neoplasia. J Clin Endocrinol Metab 53:192–199

Fox H, Sen DR (1970) A continued study of the constitutional stigmata of endometrial
adenocarcinoma. Br J Cancer 240:30–36

Frick HC, Munnell EW, Richart RM et al. (1973) Carcinoma of endometrium. Am J
Obstet Gynecol 115:663–676

Gray LA, Christopherson WM, Hoover RN (1977) Estrogen and endometrial carcinoma.
Obstet Gynecol 49:385–389

Greenblatt RB, Colle ML, Mahesh VB (1976) Ovarian and adrenal steroid production in
the postmenopausal women. Obstet Gynecol 47:383–387

Greenblatt RB, Stoddard LD (1978) The estrogen–cancer controversy. J Am Geriatr Soc
26:1–8

Greene JW (1957) Feminizing mesenchymoma with associated endometrial carcinoma.
Am J Obstet Gynecol 74:31

Grodin JM, Siiteri PK, MacDonald PC (1973) Source of estrogens production in
postmenopausal women. J Clin Endocrinol Metab 36:207–214

Gurpide E, Angers M, Vande Weile R, Lieberman S (1962) Determination of secretory
rates of estrogens in pregnant and nonpregnant women from the specific activities of
urinary metabolites. J Clin Endocrinol Metab 22:935–945

Gurpide E, Gusberg SB, Tseng L (1976) Estradiol binding and metabolism in human
endometrial hyperplasia and adenocarcinoma. J Steroid Biochem 7:891–896

Gurpide E (1978a) Metabolic influences on the action of estrogens: therapeutic applications. Pediatrics (Suppl) 62:1114–1120

Gurpide E (1978b) Enzymatic modulation of hormonal action at the target tissue. J
Toxicol Environ Health 4:249–268

Gurpide E, Marks C (1981) Influence of endometrial 17β-hydroxysteroid dehydrogenase
activity on the binding of estradiol to receptors. J Clin Endocrinol Metab 52:252–255

Gusberg SB, Kardon P (1971) Proliferative endometrial response to theca-granulosa cell
tumors. Am J Obstet Gynecol 111:633–643

Hammond GL, Nisker JA, Jones LA, Siiteri PK (1980) Estimation of the percent free
steroid in undiluted serum by centrifugal ultrafiltration-dialysis. J Biol Chem
255:5023–5026

Husslein H, Breitenecker G, Tatra G (1978) Premalignant and malignant uterine changes
in immunosuppressed renen transplant recipients. Acta Obstet Gynecol Scand
57:73–78

Hawkins RA, Oakey RE (1974) Estimation of oestrone sulfate, oestradiol-17β and oestrone in peripheral plasma: concentrations during the menstrual cycle and in men. J Endocrinol 60:3–17

Hobkirk R, Mellor JD, Nilson M (1975) In vitro metabolism of 17β-estradiol in human liver tissue. Can J Biochem 53:903–906

Horwitz RI, Feinstein AR (1978) Alternative analytic methods for case-control studies of estrogens and endometrial cancer. N Engl J Med 299:1089–1094

IARC, International Agency for Research on Cancer (1982) Caner incidence in five continents, vol IV. IARC Sci Publ 42

Jackson RL, Dockerty MB (1957) The Stein-Leventhal syndrome. Am J Obstet Gynecol 73:161–173

James VHT, Tunbridge RDG, Wilson GA et al. (1978) In: James VHT, Serio M, Giusti G (eds) The endocrine function of the human adrenal cortex. Academic, New York, p 179

Judd HL, Judd GE, Lucas WE, Yen SSC (1974) Endocrine function of the postmeno-pausal ovary: concentrations of androgens and estrogens in ovarian and peripheral vein blood. J Clin Endocrinol Metab 39:1020–1024

Judd HL, Davidson BJ, Frumar AM et al. (1980) Serum androgens and estrogens in postmenopausal women with and without endometrial cancer. Am J Obstet Gynecol 136:859–871

Kley HK, Herman J, Morgner KD, Krüskemper HL (1973) Effects of testosterone oenanthate on plasma concentrations of thyroxine, cortisol, testosterone and hormone binding proteins in patients with hypogonadism. Horm Metab Res 5:271–274

Lang JH, Wu BZ, Tang HY (1978) Endometrial carcinoma: a clinico-pathologic analysis of 108 cases. J Chin Obstet Gynecol 13:6–12

Li SY (1988) Epidemiology and etiology. In: Li SY (ed) Endometrial carcinoma. People's Medical Publishing House, Beijing, p 1–25

Longcope C (1971) Metabolic clearance and blood production rate of estrogens in postmenopausal women. Am J Obstet Gynecol 111:778–781

Longcope C, Pratt JH, Schneider SH, Fineberg SE (1976) In vitro studies on the metabolism of estrogens by muscle and adipose tissue of normal males. J Clin Endocrinol Metab 43:1134–1145

Longcope C, Pratt JH, Schneider SH, Fineberg SE (1978) Aromatization of androgens by muscle and adipose tissue in vivo. J Clin Endocrinol Metab 46:146–152

Loriaux DL, Ruder HJ, Lipsett MB (1971) The measurement of estrone sulfate in plasma. Steroids 18:463

MacDonald PC, Edman CD, Hemsell DL et al. (1978) The effect of obesity on conversion of plasma androstenedione to estrone in postmenopausal women with and without endometrial cancer. Am J Obstet Gynecol 130:448–455

Mack TM, Pike MC, Henderson BE et al. (1976) Estrogens and endometrial cancer in a retirement community. N Engl J Med 294:1262–1267

MacMahon B (1974) Risk factors for endometrial cancer. Gynecol Oncol 2:122–129

Mansell M, Hertig AT (1955) Granulosa-theca cell tumors and endometrial carcinoma. A study of their relationship and a survey of 80 cases. Obstet Gynecol 6:385

Masubuchi K, Nemoto H (1972) Epidemiologic studies on uterine cancer at Cancer Institute (Hospital), Tokyo, Cancer 30:268 – 275

Masubuchi K, Nemoto H, Masubuchi S Jr et al. (1975) Increasing incidence of endometrial carcinoma in Japan. Gynecol Oncol 3:335–346

Mattingly RF (1985) Malignant tumors of the uterus. In: Mattingly RF, Thompson JD Telinde's operative gynecology, 6th edn. Lippincott, Philadelphia, 845–876

McCarty KS Jr, Barton TK, Peete CH Jr et al. (1978) Gonadal dysgenesis with adenocarcinoma of the endometrium. An electron-microscopic and steroid receptor analysis with a review of the literature. Cancer 42:512–520

McDonald TW, Malkasian GD, Gaffcy TA (1977a) Endometrial cancer associated with feminizing tumor and polycystic ovarian disease. Obstet Gynecol 49:654–658

McDonald TW, Annegers JF, O'Fallen WM et al. (1977b) Exogenous estrogen and endometrial carcinoma: case control and incidence study. Am J Obstet Gynecol 127:572–580

Mercier C, Alfsen A, Baulieu EE (1965) Proceedings second symposium on steroid hormones, Ghent

Nimrod A, Ryan KJ (1975) Aromatization of androgens by human abdominal and breast fat tissue. J Clin Endocrinol Metab 40:367–372

Nisker JA, Hammond GL, Davidson BJ et al. (1980) Serum sex hormone binding globulin capacity and the percentage of free estradiol in postmenopausal women with and without endometrial carcinoma. Am J Obstet Gynecol 138:637–642

Norris HJ, Taylor HB (1968) Prognosis of granulosa-thecal tumor of the ovary. Cancer 21:255–263

Novak E, Yui E (1936) Relation of endometrial by hyperplasia to adenocarcinoma of the uterus. Am J Obstet Gynecol 32:674

Nunez M, Aedo AR, Landgren BM et al. (1977) Studies on the pattern of circulating steroids in the normal menstrual cycle, 6. Levels of oestrone sulphate and oestradiol sulphate. Acta Endocrinol 86:621–633

O'Brien TJ, Higashi M, Kanasugi H et al. (1982) A plasma serum estrogen-binding protein distinct from testosterone-estradiol-binding globulin. J Clin Endocrinol Metab 54:793–797

O'Dea JP, Wieland RG, Hallberg MC et al. (1979) Effect of dietary weight loss on sex steroid binding, sex steroids, and gonadotropins in obese postmenopausal women. J Lab Clin Med 93:1004–1008

Ostor AG, Fortune DW, Evans JH et al. (1978) Endometrial carcinoma in gonadal dysgenesis with and without estrogen therapy. Gynecol Oncol 6:316–327

Pack BA, Tovar R, Booth E, Brooks SC (1979) The cyclic relationship of estrogen sulfurylation to the nuclear receptor level in human endometrial curettings. J Clin Endocrinol Metab 48:420–424

Pardridge WM, Mietus LJ, Frumar AM et al. (1980) Inverse relationship between the sex hormone binding globulin level of human serum and the unidirectional clearance of testosterone and estradiol by rat brain. Am J Physiol 263:103–108

Payne AH, Lawrence CC, Foster DL, Jaffe RB (1973) Intranuclear binding of 17β-estradiol and estrone in female ovine pituitaries following incubation with oestrone sulfate. J Biol Chem 248:1598–1602

Perel E, Killinger DW (1979) The interconversion and aromatization of androgens by human adipose tissue. J Steroid Biochem 10:623–627

Raynaud JP, Mercier-Bodard C, Baulieu EE (1971) Rat estradiol binding plasma protein (EBP). Steroids 18:767

Riskallah TH, Tovell HMM, Kelly WG (1975) Production of estrone and fractional conversion of circulating androstenedione to estrone in women with endometrial carcinoma. J Clin Endocrinol Metab 40:1045–1056

Roberts KD, Rochefort JG, Bleau G, Chapdelaine A (1980) Plasma estrone sulfate levels in postmenopausal women. Steroids 35:179–187

Rodriquez J, Hart WR (1982) Endometrial cancers occurring 10 or more years after pelvic irradiation for carcinoma. Int J Gynecol Pathol 1:135–144

Rosenfield RL (1971) Plasma testosterone binding globulin and indexes of the concentration of unbound plasma androgens in normal and hirsute subjects. J Clin Endocrinol Metab 32:717

Rosenthal HE, Pietrazak E, Slaunwhite WR Jr, Sandberg AA (1972) Bonding of estrone sulfate in human plasma. J Clin Endocrinol Metab 34:805

Rosner WA (1972) A simplified method for the quantitative determination of testosterone-estradiol binding globulin activity in human plasma. J Clin Endocrinol Metab 34:983

Puder H, Corvol P, Mahoudeau JA et al. (1971) Effects of induced hyperthyrodism on steroid metabolism in man. J Clin Endocrinol Metab 33:382–387

Ruder HJ, Loriaux L, Lipsett MB (1972) Estrone sulfate: production rate and metabolism in man. J Clin Invest 51:1020–1033

Saez JM, Morera AM, Dazord A, Bertrand J (1972) Adrenal and testicular contribution to plasma estrogens. J Endocrinol 55:41–47

Sakai F, Cheix F, Clavel M et al. (1978) Increases in steroid binding globulin induced by tamoxifen in patients with carcinoma of the breast. J Endocrinol 76:219–226

Samoljik E, Santen RJ, Wells SA (1977) Adrenal suppression with aminoglutethimide. II. Differential effects of aminoglutethimide on plasma androstenedione and estrogen levels. J Clin Endocrinol Metab 45:480–487

Schindler AE, Ebert A, Fiedrick E (1972) Conversion of androstenedione to estrone by human fat tissue. J Clin Endocrinol Metab 35:627–630

Scully R (1982) Definition of endometrial carcinoma precursors. Clin Obstet Gynaecol 25:39–48

Siiteri PK, MacDonald PC (1973) Role of extraglandular estrogen in human endocrinology, In: Greep RD, Atswood EB (eds) Handbook of physiology, vol II. Williams and Wilkins, Baltimore, p 615–628

Silverberg SG, Makowski EL (1975) Endometrial carcinoma in young women taking oral contraceptive agents. Obstet Gynecol 46:503–506

Tisman G, Wu SJG (1976) Oestrogen-binding protein in blood to predict response of breast cancer to hormone manipulation. Lancet 2:145–146

Tseng L, Gurpide E (1975a) Induction of human endometrial estradiol dehydrogenase by progestins. Endocrinology 97:825–833

Tseng L, Gurpide E (1975b) Effects of progestin on estradiol receptor levels in human endometrium. J Clin Endocrinol Metab 41:402–404

Tseng L, Liu CL (1981) Stimulation of arylsulfatransferase activity by progestins in human endometrium in vitro. J Clin Endocrinol Metab 53:418–421

Van Nagell JR Jr, Roddick JW, Wallace JO (1972) Clinical correlates of endometrial carcinoma. Am J Obstet Gynecol 112:935–937

Vermeulen A, Verdonck L, Van der Straeten M, Orie N (1969) Capacity of the testosterone-binding globulin in human plasma and influence of specific binding of testosterone on its metabolic clearance rate. J Clin Endocrinol Metab 29:1470–1480

Vermeulen A (1976) The hormonal activity of the postmenopausal ovary. J Clin Endocrinol Metab 42:247–253

Vermeulen A, Verdonck L (1978) Sex hormone concentrations in postmenopausal women. Clin Endocrinol 9:59–66

Waard F de, Oettle AG (1965) A cytological survey of postmenopausal estrus in Africa. Cancer 18:450–459

Waard F de (1982) Uterine corpus. In: Schottenfeld D, Fraumeni JF (eds) Cancer epidemiology and prevention. Saunders, Philadelphia, p 901–908

Weinstein IB (1982) Carcinogenesis as a multistage process-experimental evidence. In: Bartsch H, Armstrong B (eds) Host factors in human carcinogenesis. IARC, Lyon. p 9–25

Weiss NS, Szekely DR, Austin DF (1976) Increasing incidence of endometrial cancer in the United States. N Engl J Med 294:1259–1262

Weiss NS, Sayvetz TA (1980) Incidence of endometrial cancer in relation to the use of oral contraceptives. N Engl J Med 302:551–554

Westphal U (1971) Steroid-protein interactions. Springer, Berlin Heidelberg, New York (Monographs on endocrinology, vol 4)

Wright K. Collins DC, Musey PI, Preedy JRK (1978) Specific radioimmunoassay for estrone sulfate in plasma and urine without hydrolysis. J Clin Endocrinol Metab 47:1092–1098

Wu BZ, Tang MY, Lang JH (1982) Endometrial carcinoma. In: Lin QZ (ed) Gynecologic oncology. People's Medical, Beijing, China p 85–104

Wynder EL, Escher GC, Mantel N (1966) An epidemiological investigation of cancer of the endometrium. Cancer 19:489–520

Ziel HK, Finkle WD (1975) Increased risk of endometrial carcinoma among users of conjugated estrogens. N Engl J Med 293:1167–1170

2 Pathology

Adenocarcinoma is by far the commonest primary malignancy encountered in the endometrium, arising in the glandular epithelium of the endometrium. Primary squamous cell carcinoma of the endometrium is particularly rare, and only a few cases have been reported in the world literature.

2.1 Pathologic Manifestation of Endometrial Carcinoma

2.1.1 Gross Characteristics

Endometrial carcinoma may occur in a diffuse, localized, or polypoid form.

2.1.1.1 Diffuse Carcinoma

In this form a large area of the endometrial surface, or perhaps the whole interior of the uterus, is involved. The tissue is often friable, firm, and somewhat dry and has a granular appearance.

The cancerous area is thickened and irregularly polypoid with surface ulceration and necrosis in the later stages. Necrotic foci may be yellow, gray, white, or red. In the extensive adenocarcinoma of the corpus, the disease may extend well down into the cervical canal.

Not only does the disease extend along the surface, but it also pushes into the underlying musculature. In advanced disease, the involvement may extend to the extrauterine sites and peritoneum, such as the adnexa, parametrium, bladder, and rectum (Fig. 2.1).

2.1.1.2 Localized Carcinoma

In this form the lesion seems definitely circumscribed, involving only a small area of the endometrial surface, particularly in the upper portion of the uterine cavity. The posterior wall is more likely to be involved than the anterior wall. In this form must be included a group in which the carcinoma begins in the form of a localized growth in any portion of the uterine cavity. In such instances, the surface area may remain comparatively small, although the malignant process penetrates deeply into the musculature. In the advanced stage, they may also be

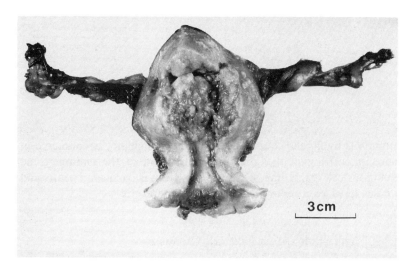

Fig. 2.1. Adenocarcinoma of the endometrium: uterine cavity filled by extensive diffuse carcinoma with cervical involvement

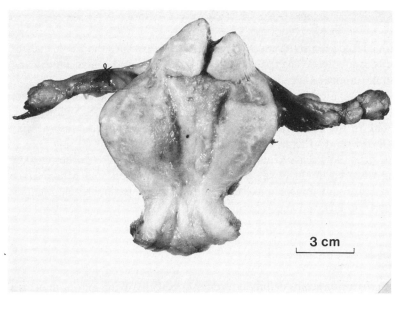

Fig. 2.2. Adenocarcinoma of the endometrium: circumscribed lesion of the posterior uterine wall with no invasion of muscle

diffuse involvement (Fig. 2.2). In the above two forms, enlargement of the uterus should be noticeable because of uterine involvement.

2.1.1.3 Polypoid Form

Cancerous tissue may be confined to a polyp which is similar to an endometrial polyp and protrudes into the uterine cavity. Neoplasm is often identified in the cornual area of the uterus. When the polyps are large, the surface may be ulcerated and necrotic, usually at the top. It is interesting to note that diagnostic curettage has, in many reported cases, apparently removed all gross trace of the lesion, so that examination of the uterus after hysterectomy shows no evidence of the disease (Fig. 2.3).

2.1.2 Microscopic Appearances

Adenocarcinoma is the commonest primary malignancy encountered in the endometrium, comprising 48.0% – 71% of carcinomas (Silverberg et al. 1972; Ng et al. 1973; Haqqani and Fox 1976; Salazar et al. 1977; Boutselis 1978; Robboy and Bradley 1979; Koss 1980; Christopherson et al. 1982). The commonest other varieties are adenoacanthoma, adenosquamous carcinoma, clear cell carcinoma, papillary adenocarcinoma, and mucinous adenocarcinoma. Primary squamous cell carcinoma of the endometrium is particularly rare (Table 2.1).

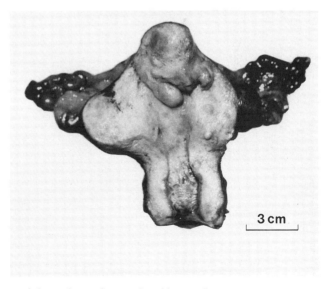

Fig. 2.3. Adenocarcinoma of the endometrium: polypoid growth pattern

Table 2.1. Histologic types of endometrial carcinoma

Series	Year	Cases	Adeno-carcinoma	Adeno-acanthoma	Adeno-squamous	Clear cell	Other
Silverberg et al.	1972	148	71 (48%)	44 (29.7%)	26 (17.6%)	7 (4.7%)	
Ng et al.	1973	542	364 (67.1%)	110 (20.3%)	68 12.6%)		
Haqqani and Fox	1976	675	69%	8%	34 (5%)		
Salazar et al.	1977	376			23%		
Boutselis	1978	586	416(67.6%)	89 (15.1%)	37 (6.3%)	8 (1.3%)	Papillary 36 (6.1%)
Robboy and Bradley	1979	–	62%	19%	11%	3%	Atypic adeno-acanthoma 4%
Koss	1980	–	65%	19%	14%	2%	
Christopherson et al.	1982	989	589 (59.6%)	215 (21.7%)	68 (6.9%)	56 (5.7%)	Papillary adenocarcinoma 46 (4.7%), secretory 15 (1.5%)

2.1.2.1 Adenocarcinoma

The glands present all degrees of departure from normal. They are increased in number and show all sorts of irregular and often bizarre convolution. The stroma is completely obliterated because of the massive hyperplasia of the glandular elements. "Back-to-back crowding" is formed. The size of the glands is variable within a given neoplasm and also varies from one cancer to another. There may be infolding of the lining epithelium into the gland lumens, which in other neoplasms is evidence of a papilliferous growth. Rarely gland formation is inconspicuous. The cells are enlarged, often pseudostratified, and have enlarged nuclei which occur at varying levels within the epithelium. The nuclear chromatin is clumped and mitoses are variable in frequency. Lipid-laden macrophages are often observed in the stroma particularly in the more differentiated cancer. Necrosis, hemorrhage, and the formation of psammoma may occur. Marked reactive inflammatory infiltration with round cells and leukocytes can usually be seen (Fig. 2.4).

2.1.2.2 Adenoacanthoma

Adenocarcinoma coexisting with benign-appearing squamous epithelium is designated adenoacanthoma. The squamous component may be localized and is

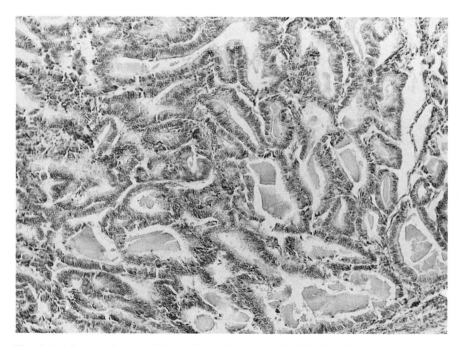

Fig. 2.4. Adenocarcinoma of the endometrium: grade I. H & E, × 40

more commonly multicentric in its distribution. The squamous epithelium may have the varying degrees of metaplasia, the squamous cells are mature and well differentiated, and the acanthosis and keratin may be prominent in some neoplasms. Because poorly differentiated glandular epithelium and squamous epithelium grow in solid sheets or nests, the distinction between them may be difficult on light microscopy. In view of the evidence obtained by ultrastructural studies, these two elements are readily identified by the different characteristics of the cell surfaces and their cytoplasmic organelles (Fig. 2.5).

2.1.2.3 Adenosquamous Carcinoma

Neoplasms having both a malignant glandular and squamous component are designated adenosquamous carcinoma. The squamous component may occur in juxtaposition to the glandular component or may be intermingled with the neoplastic glands. Silverberg et al. (1972) and Ng et al. (1973) described that in 60% of cases the glandular component is dominant while the squamous epithelium is equally prominent in 40% of the cases. In 80% of the cases, the squamous epithelium is reminiscent of that associated with the large cell type of cervical squamous carcinoma; in 16% it was characterized by the presence of

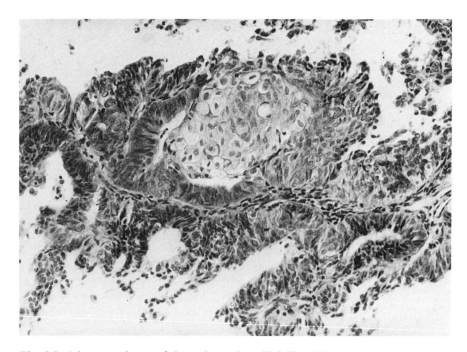

Fig. 2.5. Adenoacanthoma of the endometrium. H & E, × 100

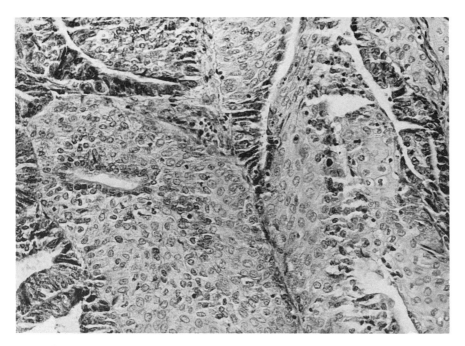

Fig. 2.6. Adenosquamous carcinoma of the endometrium. H & E, × 100

keratin; and in 4% it resembled the small cell type of cancer observed in the uterine cervix. The glandular component was well differentiated in 13.6% of cases, moderately differentiated in 57.6%, and poorly differentiated in 28.8%. The prognosis is closely related to the degree of differentiation of the glandular component and is, therefore, worse than that for pure adenocarcinoma or adenoacanthoma (Fig. 2.6).

2.1.2.4 Clear Cell Carcinoma

The lesion consists of hobnail or flattened cells with a clear cytoplasm. The cells are arranged in solid masses or are characterized by papillary, tubular, or cystic patterns. With PAS stains there is evidence of diastase-digestible glycogen in the cytoplasm of the neoplastic cells. Kurman and Scully (1976) recorded 21 such cases, many of which showed both a clear cell and a tubular pattern, with psammoma bodies in a few cases. The neoplasms are thought to be of mullerian rather than mesonephric origin (Fig. 2.7). The clinical stage at diagnosis is somewhat more advanced. The prognosis of this lesion seems to be very poor (Christopherson et al. 1982).

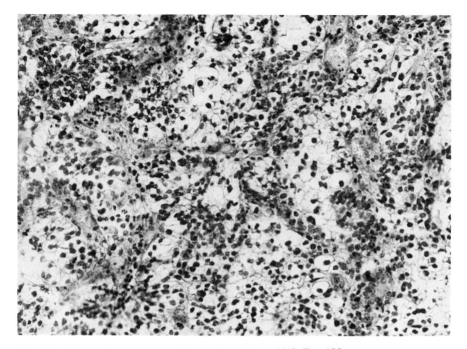

Fig. 2.7. Clear cell carcinoma of the endometrium. H & E, × 100

2.1.2.5 Pipillary Carcinoma (Fig. 2.8)

Papillary carcinoma is distinguished from papillary clear cell carcinoma by the absence of a significant clear cell component. The cells have sparse, basophilic, or amphophilic cytoplasm and are PAS negative.

Papillary carcinoma of the endometrium is distinctly uncommon and until recently had been largely unstudied. Chen et al. (1985) suggested that two clinicopathologic varieties of papillary neoplasia with different prognostic implications could be distinguished: papillary serous carcinoma and papillary adenocarcinoma. Uterine papillary serous carcinomas resemble papillary serous carcinoma of the ovary or fallopian tube, displaying a complex papillary architecture with fibrovascular stalks covered with irregular stratified and tufted malignant epithelial cells. The cells have a high nuclear/cytoplasmic ratio and may be markedly pleomorphic. Many have anaplastic, hyperchromatic nuclei, sometimes with prominent nucleoli. Macronuclei are seen occasionally. Mitoses are numerous and may be atypical. Psammoma bodies are sometimes present. Epithelial borders tend to be uneven due to epithelial tufting and variation in the size and shape of the neoplastic cells.

In papillary adenocarcinoma, the epithelium is pseudostratified and composed of more uniform columnar cells without the anaplasia seen in the papillary serous tumors. Some mitoses are present, but these are generally not atypical and

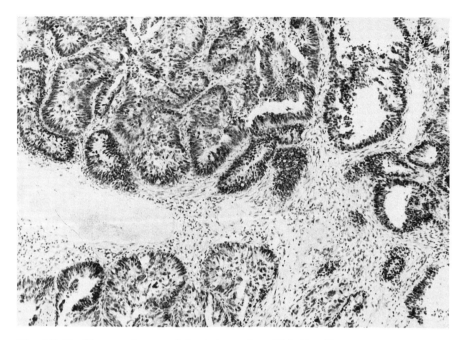

Fig. 2.8. Papillary carcinoma of the endometrium. H & E, × 40

macronucleoli and psammoma bodies are not present. The irregular tufting seen in serous tumors is also absent. Some cells had small- to intermediate-sized nucleoli.

Papillary serous endometrial carcinomas are characterized by an unusually high risk of recurrence and death. Survival in papillary serous carcinomas is worse than in nonpapillary adenocarcinoma (Hendrickson et al. 1982; Chen et al. 1985). Jeffrey et al. (1986) reported that 86.7% of patients with papillary serous tumors in all stages suffered recurrence and that 73.3% died from the disease.

2.1.2.6 Secretory Adenocarcinoma

The neoplastic cells are arranged in glandular patterns. The glands are lined by cells with uniform subnuclear vacuolization reminiscent of that observed in the immediate postovulatory period of a normal menstrual cycle (Hertig and Gore 1960; Kurman and Scully 1976). The morphologic changes are sometimes encountered in a well-differentiated endometrial adenocarcinoma and may coexist with a normal endometrium, reflecting a progesterone effect. There is still controversy on the nature of secretory adenocarcinoma. Some authors maintain that this is not a specific form of endometrial cancer but a feature which may exist focally or diffusely in another typical well-differentiated endometrial adeno-

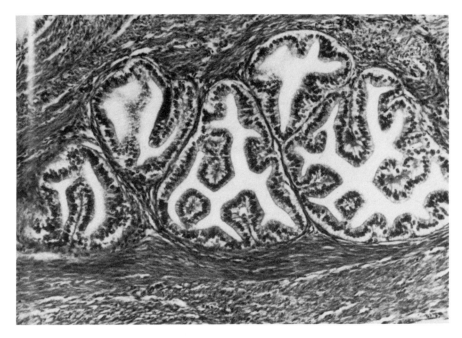

Fig. 2.9. Well-differentiated secretory carcinoma of the endometrium. (Adapted from Christopherson et al. 1982) H & E, × 79

carcinoma. Some authors consider that this is a form of clear cell carcinoma (Kay 1957; Silverberg and DeGiorgi 1973) (Fig. 2.9).

2.1.3 Histologic Grade

The histologic grading of endometrial carcinoma provides important information about the biologic potential of the neoplasm. In general, the higher the grade, the worse the prognosis but the greater the radiosensitivity. Thus grading is most important for prognosis and occasionally for determining the type of treatment. Originally Broders (1925) classified endometrial carcinoma into four grades by degree of differentiation:

Grade 1: Well-differentiated, undifferentiated cells are less than 25%, glands are increased in number, and "back-to-back crowding" is formed. The stroma is rarefied and focally scant.

Grade 2: Undifferentiated cells are less than 50%, and glandular epithelium proliferates and may grow into the lumen in a papillary fashion. The size and position of nuclei are inconstant.

Grade 3: Undifferentiated cells are less than 75%, glandular epithelium proliferates obviously. The epithelium forming small acini is stratified.

Grade 4: Undifferentiated cells are from 75% to 100%. The glandular structure is completely obliterated.

The neoplasms are divided into three grades in FIGO staging of endometrial carcinoma.

I   Highly differentiated adenomatous carcinomas
II   Differentiated adenomatous carcinomas with partly solid areas
III Predominantly solid or entirely undifferentiated carcinomas

The Broders' method is seldom used because it is difficult and time-consuming and, furthermore, there is marked individual variation in assessing grades 2 and 3, because the criteria are ill defined. Comparing the Broders' classification and the FIGO grading (FIGO 1970), grade I FIGO grading might combine Broders' grade 1 and 2, and grade II and III FIGO grading might correspond to grades 3 and 4 of Broders' classification respectively. If the grade of a given carcinoma varies in different portions of the tumor, the tumor is graded by its most malignant portion. Sections used for grading should be of reasonable size and from different areas of the tumor. Basically, grading is based on the extirpated uterus, and the curettage sample could be used only for the patients with primary radiotherapy or preoperative radiotherapy.

Distribution of the glandular component in different types of endometrial carcinoma was different. In adenocarcinoma and adenoacanthoma, the glandular component was well or moderately differentiated; and in contrast to adenocarcinoma and adenoacanthoma the glandular component of the adenosquamous carcinoma was somewhat less differentiated. Table 2.2 shows that more than 80% of the glandular components in adenocarcinoma and adenoacanthoma were grade I or II, but in adenosquamous carcinoma more than 80% of glandular components were grade II or III.

Table 2.2. Histologic grading of glandular components in different histologic types of endometrial carcinoma. (Adapted from Reagan 1981, p. 546)

Histologic types	Total (n)	Grades							
		I		II		III		IV	
		(n)	(%)	(n)	(%)	(n)	(%)	(n)	(%)
Adenocarcinoma	367	141	38.4	160	43.6	55	15.0	11	3.0
Adenoacanthoma	141	52	36.9	73	51.8	13	9.2	3	2.1
Adenosquamous carcinoma	107	14	13.1	62	57.9	28	26.2	3	2.8
Total	615	207	33.6	295	48.0	96	15.6	17	2.8

2.1.4 Pattern of Spread

In general impression, endometrial carcinoma is frequently a "surface rider." It is much less prone to local or lymphatic extension than cervical malignancy.

The dissemination of endometrial carcinoma is through the lymphatics, direct extension, transtubal spread, peritoneal implantation, or blood vascular metastasis. In many cases, more than one route is involved in the dissemination of the disease (Fig. 2.10).

2.1.4.1 Lymphatic Spread

According to Henriksen (1949), there are three main lymphatic channels draining the uterine corpus. One channel drains the lower and midportion of the uterus and is similar to that from the cervix. This includes the paracervical, parametrial, obturator, hypogastric, external iliac, common iliac, sacral, inguinal, and paraaortic lymph nodes. The second channel draining the upper portion of the uterus, like those of the tube and ovary, directly drains into the aortic nodes. The third channel draining the fundus of uterus follows the course of the round ligament to the deep and superficial inguinal nodes.

Of the 64 cases of endometrial carcinoma at autopsy studied by Henriksen (1949), lymph node spread in each clinical stage and different groups of lymph

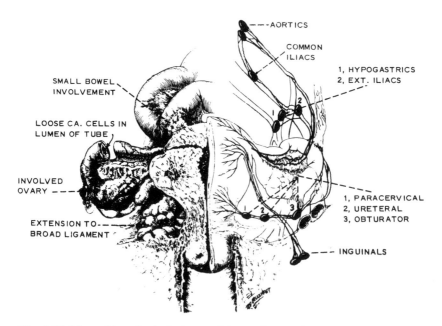

Fig. 2.10. Normal lymphatic drainage of the uterine corpus and the sites of local pelvic extension of endometrial carcinoma. (Adapted from DiSaia PJ et al. 1975)

nodes was as follows: in 1 of 8 the cases of clinical stage I, in 10 of 18 the cases of clinical stage II, in 38 of the 38 cases with advanced stage; in 41% of the cases with involvement of the parametrial lymph nodes, in 32% of the cases with involvement of sacral, common iliac, and inguinal and aortic lymph nodes, in 36% of the cases with metastases of paracervical, hypogastric, obturator and external iliac lymph nodes, and in 17% of the cases with metastases of the inguinal lymph nodes (Fig. 2.11).

Morrow et al. (1973), in a review of 15 years literature on pelvic lymphadenectomy in endometrial carcinoma, noted that approximately 10.6% of (369/454 cases) stage I disease had metastases to the pelvic nodes and 36.5% (31/85 cases) of stage II carcinoma had one or more pelvic nodes involved. A definite correlation between lymph gland involvement and invasion of cervix was observed.

The information gained from pelvic lymphadenectomy studies also indicated that the incidence of pelvic node metastasis increased when the tumor was more advanced and more undifferentiated.

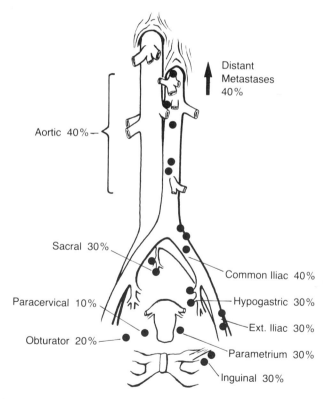

Fig. 2.11. Incidence of lympth node involvement in endometrial carcinoma. (Adapted from Henriksen 1949)

2.1.4.2 Cervical Involvement

Involvement of the cervix in endometrial carcinoma infers an increased possibility of lymph node involvement with a worse prognosis. There is a considerable variation in the reported frequency of cervical involvement in endometrial carcinoma, ranging from 3% to 24% (Kottmeier 1973; Homesley et al. 1977; Boutselis 1978). Among the 7561 patients reported in 17 individual studies cited by Rutledge, there were 881 patients or 11.6% with cervical involvement (Rutledge 1974). The criteria of cervical involvement should be standardized.

2.1.4.3 Myometrial Invasion

Myometrium is the major invasive location in the dissemination of endometrial carcinoma. The depth of myometrial invasion is associated with the other poor prognosis factors, poor differentiation and lymph node involvement. The deeper the myometrial invasion, the worse the prognosis. This is especially true if the myometrial invasion involves the outer half of the uterine wall. The nearer the invasion to the serosal surface of the uterus, the lower the eventual survival (Frick et al. 1973; Jones 1975; Lutz et al. 1978; Connelly et al. 1982).

Reagan and Fu (1981) reported that, in 362 endometrial carcinomas, the neoplasm was confined to the endometrium in 200 or 55.2% of cases. Penetration of the myometrium up to one-half its thickness was present in 96 or 26.5% of the cases. In 39 or 10.8% of the cases, there was invasion to a level which exceeded one-half the thickness of the myometrium and in 27 or 7.5% of the cases there was spread beyond the limits of the uterus.

In a series of 191 stage I endometrial carcinomas, in 155 or 81% of the cases the neoplasm was confined to the endometrium and infiltrated up to one-half the thickness of the myometrium. The neoplasm penetrated more than one-half the thickness of the myometrium in 36 or 19% of the cases (Li 1988). The depth of myometrial invasion may severely influence the eventual prognosis. So the myometrial penetration should be carefully considered in making a schedule for treatment.

2.1.4.4 Transtubal Spread

Spread by a transtubal route may be the main route of cancer cells to the pelvic and abdominal cavity. Dahle (1956) reported that cancer was identified in the tubal lumens in 22 (or 34%) of 65 patients with endometrial carcinoma studied at autopsy. This is compatible with the reported frequency of cancer cells observed in the cul-de-sac of women with endometrial carcinoma, which would support the fact that transtubal spread is the main route of cancer cells to the pelvic and abdominal cavity.

2.1.4.5 Pelvic or Extrapelvic Spread

The dissemination of carcinoma in the pelvic cavity is through the lymphatics, and hematogenous and direct extension. In advanced stages, the disease may extend to the extrapelvic sites, and distant metastases may also occur.

Sites of pelvic involvement include the cervix, vagina, vulva ovaries, fallopian tubes, parametrium, pelvic peritoneum, urethra, bladder, ureters, and lymph nodes. The liver, bowel, lung, bone, adrenal, kidney, pancreas, and spleen are frequently reported to be the extrapelvic sites. Plentl and Friedman (1971) reported that the lung (8.3%) is the commonest site for distant metastases, followed by the liver (5.9%) and bone (3.4%). Aalders et al. in 1984 reviewed 83 cases of endometrial carcinoma with stage IV from 1960 to 1977 (at the Norwegian Radium Hospital); 36% of the cases had pulmonary metastases, 23% of the cases had, metastases to multiple sites, and metastases to the lymph nodes and bladder were found in 13%. In one study of 26 cases of endometrial carcinoma 50% had stage IV metastases of the lymph nodes, and involvement of multiple sites was observed in 15.5%. The distribution of distant metastases in endometrial carcinoma is shown in Fig. 2.12.

In studies based on autopsied cases, death was attributable to cancer or complications of therapy in 77.7%–85.3% of cases (Beck and Latour 1963; Henriksen 1949). In one study, death was attributable to uremia or pyelo-nephritis in 25.3%, to hemorrhage or cachexia in 17.4%, to carcinomatosis in 15.8%, to pulmonary emboli or thrombosis in 14.2%, and to peritonitis and intestinal obstruction in 12.6% of the cases. In 14.7%–22.3% of the cases, death was attributable to factors unrelated to the presence of endometrial carcinoma (Reagan and Fu 1981).

2.2 Ultrastructural, Chromosomal Karyotyping, and Nuclear DNA Studies

2.2.1 Ultrastructural Studies

To distinguish poorly differentiated glandular epithelium from squamous epithelium may be difficult on light microscopy because both grow in solid sheets or nests. These two elements are readily identified by the different characteristics of the cell surface and their cytoplasmic organelles using electronmicroscopy. Squamous cells can be recognized by numerous desmosomes between the neighboring cells and the lack of a luminal formation. In the cytoplasm, abundant tonofilaments are present. In the keratinizing variant, tonofilaments form coarse, dense aggregates. Keratohyaline granules are sometimes present. Rough endoplasmic reticulum and Golgi membranes are poorly developed and few in number. The cells having a clear cytoplasm contain multiple aggregates of glycogen. The nuclei of the malignant squamous cells exhibit invaginations and convolutions. The chromatin aggregates are irregular in size and shape. Nucleoli are often identified. At the junction with the stroma, the basal lamina is

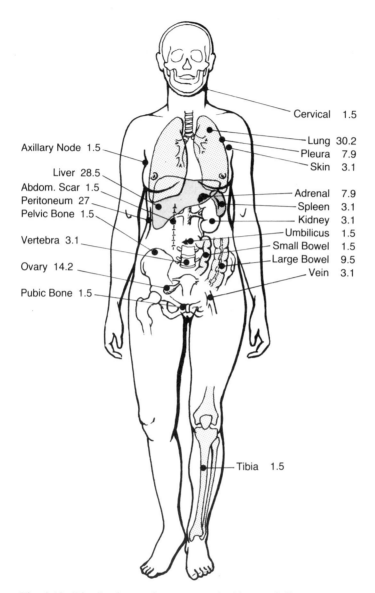

Fig. 2.12. Distribution and percentage incidence of distant metastases in endometrial carcinoma. (Adapted from Henriksen 1949)

incomplete or lacking. Cytoplasmic processes extend into the stroma. These features indicate the invasive behavior. Benign-appearing squamous cells have a smooth regular nuclear configuration, uniform chromatin, and intact basal lamina (Fig. 2.13).

Glandular cells exhibit a luminal formation lined with abundant microvilli. Desmosomal junctions are few in number. The cytoplasmic organelle consists of

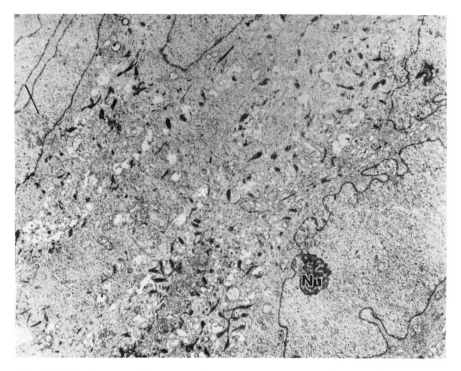

Fig. 2.13. Electrophotomicrograph of squamous component in an adenosquamous carcinoma. The cells are jointed by numerous desmosomes. Tonofilaments are abundant. Rough endoplasmic reticulum and Golgi membranes are few in number. Note convoluted nuclear envelope and nucleolus (*Nu*). (Adapted from Reagan and Fu 1981), × 7650

profiles of rough endoplasmic reticulum, well-developed Golgi membranes, vacuoles, and scattered ribosomes. Glycogen particles are sometimes present. Mucinous vacuoles are rarely identified. In the well-differentiated glandular neoplasms, a columnar or cuboidal configuration is maintained and the cytoplasmic organelles are arranged in orderly fashion.

In the poorly differentiated glandular tumors, the cytoplasmic organelles are disorganized. Small, irregular, slit-like glandular lumens have microvilli projecting into them. Bundles of microfilaments with a thickness of 80–100 Å may be present but tonofilaments are scant or absent (Fig. 2.14), (Ferenczy and Richart 1974).

The abundant accumulation of glycogen particles and lipid droplets are the characteristics of clear cell adenocarcinoma. These are related to the clear cytoplasmic appearance. Rough endoplasmic reticulum and Golgi membranes are abundant. In cells having granular cytoplasm, mitochondria are more numerous than in the clear cells. Electron-dense membrane-bound bodies with a crystalline appearance are sometimes observed. The microvilli are short, few in number, and irregular in space. The above characteristics are unlike those seen in

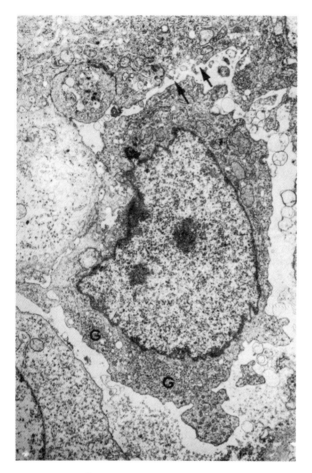

Fig. 2.14. Electrophotomicrograph of clear cell adenocarcinoma. Glycogen particles (*G*) are abundant. Microvilli (*arrows*) are short and few in number. (Reagan and Fu 1981), ×6750

the clear cell variant of renal cell carcinoma and support a müllerian rather than mesonephric origin for the clear cell carcinomas of the female genital tract.

2.2.2 Chromosomal Karyotyping and Nuclear DNA Studies

Diploid or near diploid chromosome counts in the majority of cases have been demonstrated by chromosome karyotyping of endometrial carcinoma (Hertig and Gore 1960; Katayama and Jones 1967; Stanley and Kirkland 1968; Tseng and Jones 1969; Granberg et al. 1974; Atkin 1976). Hertig and Gore (1960) and Stanley and Kirkland (1968) reported that the chromosome number is less frequently high. Atkin (1976) reported that 73% of 181 endometrial adeno-carcinomas have less than 55 chromosomes or an equivalent nuclear DNA content. Twenty-seven percent had a higher ploidy level. Correlation between the ploidy level and the degree of differentiation and prognosis has been demonstrated. In 181 patients with endometrial carcinoma, 93% of well-differentiated neoplasms, 69% of moderate-differentiated neoplasms, and 59% of poorly differentiated neoplasms had a near-diploid mode respectively. Patients with near-diploid neoplasms were found to have a 5-year survival rate of 77% in contrast to 22% of patients with higher ploidy neoplasms.

Reagan and Fu (1981) reported that there are significant differences in nuclear DNA between endometrial adenoacanthomas and adenosquamous carcinomas. Adenoacanthomas have near-diploid stem cell lines for both glandular and squamous components. In adenosquamous carcinomas the glandular cells had hyperploid stem cell lines. The squamous components had either the same hyperploid distribution as the glandular cells or peritetraploid stem cell lines. The higher ploidy level observed in the glandular component of adenosquamous carcinoma may partly explain the poor prognosis of adenosquamous carcinoma.

In nuclear DNA studies on endometrial adenocarcinoma, it was also found that adenocarcinoma having high ploidy levels show a poorer prognosis than those having near-diploid nodes.

2.3 Rare Types of Endometrial Carcinoma

2.3.1 Argyrophil Cell Carcinoma or Small Cell Carcinoma

The existence of primary carcinoids and neuroendocrine carcinoma of the uterine cervix has been widely recognized (Tateishi et al. 1975; Albores-Saavedra et al. 1976; Albores-Saavedra et al. 1979; Pazdur et al. 1981). However, endometrial carcinoma with neuroendocrine features, i.e., argyrophil cell carci-noma or small cell carcinoma, has rarely been described in the literature. Up to 1986, only five case reports in English have described small cell endometrial carcinomas containing neurosecretory-type granules (Table 2.3) (Olson et al. 1982; Bannatyne et al. 1983; Kumar 1984; Paz et al. 1985; Tohya et al. 1986). Olson et al. (1982) described that endometrial small cell carcinoma contains neurosecretory granules and suggested the possibility that this neoplasm might arise from the neuroendocrine cell system. Feyrter (1938) described that these neoplasms appear to arise from cells of the diffuse epithelial endocrine cell system. However, this concept has recently been criticized due to the coexistence of neuroendocrine carcinoma with conventional carcinoma in the uterine cervix (Mullins et al. 1981). Ueda et al. (1978, 1979) and Prade et al. (1982) demonstrated neurosecretory granules and the argyrophilic cells in the usual type of endo-metrial carcinoma, endeavoring to show that the presence of argyrophilic cells is common. Histochemical and immunohistochemical evidence has also accumu-lated in support of the concept that small cell carcinoma may arise from

Table 2.3. Reported cases of small cell carcinoma of the endometrium

Series	Year	Age (years)	Symptoms	Pathology	Argyrophilia	Dense-core granules by electron microscopy
Olson et al.	1982	60	Metrorrhagia	Large uterine corpus tumor, perforating left cornu and lower uterine segment, metastases in regional nodes	Negative	Yes
Bannatyne et al.	1983	–	–	Uterine corpus tumor, metastases in regional nodes	Negative	Yes
Kumar	1984	23	Metrorrhagia	Uterine corpus tumor, extending into serosa, metastases to ovaries, peritoneum and bone marrow	Negative	Yes
Paz et al.	1985	59	Metrorrhagia	Tumor limited to body of endometrial polyp	Positive	Yes
Tohya et al.	1986	64	Abdominal vaginal cytology	Large uterine corpus tumor, extending into serosa, metastases to vaginal wall	Negative, vaginal tumor positive	Yes

epithelial precursors and not from the neuroendocrine cell system (Aguirre et al. 1983; Inoue et al. 1984). Moreover, the existence and histogenesis of such neoplasms remain rather controversial.

Pearse (1969, 1974) introduced the concept of APUD (amine precursor uptake and decarboxylation) cells to characterize a variety of neuroendocrine cells which are of neural crest origin and share a number of electron microscopic and cytochemical characteristics. Some studies revealed that the patients with endometrial argyrophil cell carcinoma tended to be associated more frequently with obesity, hypertension, and diabetes mellitus than those with the usual endometrial carcinoma.

Calcitonin is also found in the tumor cells, which suggests the possibility of other polypeptide hormone production related directly to the above-stated complications, obesity, hypertension, and diabetes mellitus, because the production of calcitonin is intimately related with that of parathyroid hormone, subunit of the glycoprotein hormones and adrenocorticotropic hormone (ACTH) in various tumors (Rosen and Weintraub 1974; Coombes et al. 1976).

2.3.2 Primary Pure Squamous Cell Carcinoma of the Endometrium

A primary endometrial malignancy purely squamous in nature is extremely rare. Kay (1978) supported the criteria of diagnosis for pure squamous endometrial carcinoma previously suggested by Fluhmann (1928):

1. There is no coexisting endometrial adenocarcinoma.
2. Primary squamous carcinoma of the cervix is absent.
3. If in situ squamous cancer in the cervix is noted, no connection exists between it and the endometrial squamous tumor.
4. No connection between the endometrial tumor and the squamous epithelium of the cervix is found.

Of the 21 cases reported since 1887, only 17 have been documented adequately enough to test against the criteria (Fluhmann 1928; Hopkin et al. 1970; Gompel and Silverberg 1976; Kay 1978; Melin et al. 1979; Bibbo et al. 1980).

Squamous elements in the endometrium are thought to arise from metaplasia of reverse stem or totipotential cells that lie between the columnar epithelium and glandular basement membrane (Fluhmann 1928; Baggish and Woodruff 1967; Kay 1978). Factors implicated in the development of squamous metaplasia include pyometra, foreign irritants, vitamin A deficiency, and senile involution (Fluhmann 1928; Hopkin et al. 1970; Gompel and Silverberg 1976; Kay 1978).

Squamous carcinoma may arise from a normal endometrium and prior benign squamous change is apparently not needed. However, pyometra has been found in about half of these women (Hopkin et al. 1970; Kay 1978). Although the exact relationship is not clear, it is tempting to speculate that the pyometra and attendant squamous metaplasia preceded the malignant squamous lesion.

2.4 Endometrial Hyperplasia and Adenocarcinoma in Situ

Distinguishing between hyperplasia and adenocarcinoma is based mainly on the pathologic diagnosis. Unfortunately this is not a simple question, because its complexity has been compounded by the lack of uniform terminology and the imprecision of definitions. Thomas Cullon, in his book *Cancer of the Uterus* published in 1900, stated that there was close association between hyperplasia and adenocarcinoma of the endometrium, and endometrial atypical hyperplasia could be considered the premalignant stage of endometrial carcinoma. Taylor (1932) and Novak and Yui (1936) documented his hypothesis. Gusburg in 1947 reported the relationship between adenomatous hyperplasia and endogenous, exogenous estrogens and pointed out that actual carcinomatous changes could occur in adenomatous hyperplasia. Hertig et al. (1949) first suggested the classification of endometrial hyperplasia and called the endometrial atypical hyperplasia carcinoma in situ of the endometrium. Campbell and Barter (1961) classified endometrial hyperplasia into three grades.

The association of hyperplasia with adenocarcinoma of the endometrium has been amply documented (Bamforth 1956; Campbell and Barter 1961; Gray et al. 1974). Both are associated with estrogen. However, it is more difficult to prove that hyperplasia is a transitional stage (Benjamin and Block 1977; Rosenwaks et al. 1979).

2.4.1 Classification of Endometrial Hyperplasia

2.4.1.1 Classification of Glandular Intraepithelial Neoplasia

In 1974, Vellions commented that the so-called hyperplasia of the endometrium would be more appropriately termed "dysplasias," in a manner analogous to lesions of the cervix. Richart (1973) developed the unifying concept of cervical intraepithelial neoplasia (CIN) to simplify and clarify the diagnostic and therapeutic aspects of premalignant cervical lesions. Ruffolo et al. (1983) proposed a classification of endometrial hyperplasias analogous to CIN of the cervix, termed "glandular intraepithelial neoplasia" (GIN). Such a concept seems likely to be acceptable to both gynecologists and pathologists in view of the general acceptance of the concept of cervical intraepithelial neoplasia by both groups. The correlation between the classification of GIN and existing terminologies is shown in Table 2.4. GIN I includes cystic hyperplasia and adenomatous hyperplasia without atypia. GIN II includes adenomatous hyperplasia to a moderate degree and atypical hyperplasia.

GIN III includes marked adenomatous hyperplasia, severe atypical hyperplasia, and carcinoma in situ. The likelihood of progression of the various grades of GIN can be estimated from various reports. Sherman (1978) studied 204 patients and concluded that patients with GIN I have a 20% chance of developing invasive carcinoma 2–10 years later, while for those with GIN II and GIN III the figure was the same. 57%.

Table 2.4. Classifications of hyperplasia of the endometrium

	Year	GIN I	GIN II	GIN III
Campbell and Barter	1961	Benign hyperplasia Atypical hyperplasia	Atypical hyperplasia Type II Type II	Atypical hyperplasia type III
Beutler et al.	1963	Cystic proliferation and glandular hyperplasia		Glandular hyperplasia with atypical epithelial proliferation
Gusberg and Kaplan	1963	Mild adenomatous hyperplasia	Moderate adenomatous hyperplasia	Marked adenomatous hyperplasia
Gore and Hertig	1966	Cystic hyperplasia and adenomatous hyperplasia	Anaplasia	Carcinoma in situ
Vellios	1972	Cystic hyperplasia and adenomatous hyperplasia	Atypical hyperplasia	Carcinoma in situ
Poulsen and Taylor	1975	Cystic hyperplasia and adenomatous hyperplasia	Adenomatous hyperplasia	Atypical hyperplasia

2.4.1.2 Histologic Classification

Four forms of endometrial hyperplasia may be recognized histologically (Fox 1983):

1. Cystic glandular hyperplasia
2. Adenomatoid hyperplasia
3. Glandular hyperplasia with architectural atypia
4. Glandular hyperplasia with cytologic atypia, which is synonymous with the term "atypical hyperplasia."

2.4.2 Pathology of Endometrial Hyperplasia

2.4.2.1 Cystic Glandular Hyperplasia (Fig. 2.15)

Cystic glandular hyperplasia involves the entire endometrium, which is thick-ened and polypoid and is often characterized by a velvety appearance; tiny cysts may be seen. The myometrium is also hypertrophied, and the uterus is bulky. Under microscopic manifestation, there is diffuse involvement of the endo-metrium, and the distinction between the functional and basal zones is lost. The glands are characterized by their marked variability in size – some large, others normal, and still others unusually small. The glands retain their regular, smooth, and rounded outline. The surface epithelium and the cells lining the gland lumens may be columnar, cuboidal, or flattened. The nuclei of the columnar cells are elongated, usually vesicular, and are oriented perpendicular to the surface. Pseudostratification, if present, is patchy and minimal.

Mitoses in both stroma and glands are variable but may usually be found without much difficulty. Atypical mitoses are not encountered. The ratio of stroma to glands is normal, since the stroma shares in the hyperplastic process and usually appears markedly cellular. The morphology has led to the term "Swiss cheese hyperplasia."

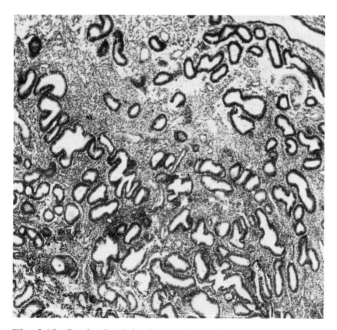

Fig. 2.15. Cystic glandular hyperplasia of endometrium. H & E, × 40

2.4.2.2 Adenomatoid Hyperplasia (Fig. 2.16)

Adenomatoid hyperplasia is a rare lesion and invariably focal in nature. It is characterized by a simple excess of glands of normal shape and approximately normal size, with a marked reduction in the intervening stroma. There is no cellular atypia, and its appearance differs from that of a normal proliferative endometrium only by the abundance of glands and the striking reduction of intervening stroma.

2.4.2.3 Glandular Hyperplasia with Architectural Atypia (Fig. 2.17)

Glandular hyperplasia with architectural atypia is restricted to the glandular component of the endometrium and is usually focal. The glands, although variable in size, are often rather larger than normal and are more numerous, the intervening stroma being reduced. There is an abnormal pattern of glandular growth, with outpouchings or buddings, of the glandular epithelium into the stroma and pseudopapillary projections of epithelium into the glandular lumen. The glands are lined with regular, darkly staining, cuboid cells with rounded central nuclei. There is no cellular or nuclear atypia and little stratification. Mitotic figures may be present and are of normal form.

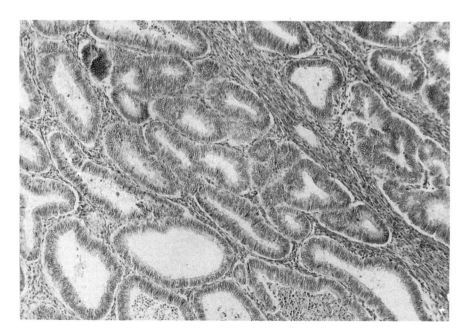

Fig. 2.16. Adenomatoid hyperplasia of endometrium. H & E, × 100

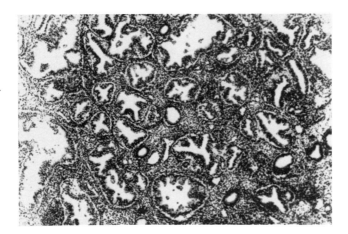

Fig. 2.17. Glandular hyperplasia of endometrium with architectural atypia. (Adapted from Fox 1983) H & E, × 30

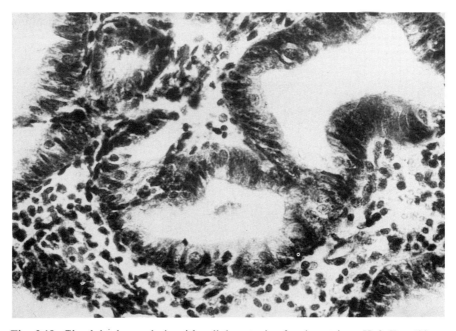

Fig. 2.18. Glandular hyperplasia with cellular atypia of endometrium. H & E, × 400

2.4.2.4 Glandular Hyperplasia with Cellular Atypia (Fig. 2.18)

Glandular hyperplasia with cellular atypia is also restricted to the endometrial glands and always appears to be focal in nature. Sometimes it is multifocal, and this may give a false impression of diffuse involvement. However, the foci of glands with cellular atypia are always separated from each other either by normal glands or by glands showing another variety of endometrial hyperplasia. In the affected areas of the endometrium, there is a marked reduction in stroma, and the glands either show a "back-to-back" manifestation or are separated from each other only by narrow bands of stroma. The glands are often markedly irregular in shape and size, showing a degree of generalized irregularity and deformity. The cells lining the glands show varying degrees of cellular and · nuclear atypia such as nuclear crowding, multilayering, intraluminal tufting, and mitotic activity. The nuclei are generally small, and all mitotic figures are normal. The intraluminal epithelial tufts may appear to fuse with each other to give a cribriform appearance, and these apparent "bridges" retain a stromal support. The cytoplasm is usually relatively scanty and amphophilic, but in some instances with the most severe cellular atypia it may be abundant and markedly eosinophilic.

This form of hyperplasia is commonly classified as mild, moderate, or severe. The degree of cellular and nuclear atypia may vary not only from one area to another but even within the same gland. Sometimes it is very difficult to differentiate between a glandular hyperplasia with severe cellular atypia and a well-differentiated adenocarcinoma.

2.4.3 Relationships of Various Forms of Endometrial Hyperplasia

It is certain that various types of hyperplasia coexisting in the same endometrium may be seen. Cystic glandular hyperplasia is frequently found in pure form but is not uncommonly seen in combination with glandular hyperplasia and architectural atypia or cellular atypia. There is often an accompanying glandular hyperplasia with architectural atypia and cystic glandular hyperplasia or glandular hyperplasia with cellular atypia. A pure glandular hyperplasia with architectural atypia is not uncommon, but it is relatively uncommon to encounter glandular hyperplasia with cellular atypia in isolated form. The only exception to this general rule of frequent coexistence is adenomatoid hyperplasia, which always appears to develop in an otherwise normal endometrium.

The relationships of various forms of endometrial hyperplasia may suggest that the various forms of hyperplasia are different morphologic expressions of a common basic abnormality of growth or that they form a continuous spectrum.

2.4.4 Etiology and Pathogenesis of Endometrial Hyperplasia

It is generally accepted that all forms of endometrial hyperplasia, with the possible exception of adenomatoid hyperplasia, may be caused by prolonged unopposed estrogenic stimulation of the endometrium. Unopposed estrogen may originate from an anovulatory cycle, an estrogenic ovarian tumor, or the administration of exogenous estrogens. It is almost certainly the case that the endometrium which is subjected to prolonged estrogenic stimulation will eventually develop some degree of cystic glandular hyperplasia. Glandular hyperplasia with either architectural or cellular atypical hyperplasia usually coexists with a cystic glandular hyperplasia. However, glandular hyperplasia is always focal rather than diffuse and is sometimes found as a localized lesion in an otherwise normal or atrophic endometrium. Therefore, it seems reasonable to suggest that these forms of hyperplasia represent a local tissue abnormality, which can be independent of estrogenic stimulation but is more commonly estrogen induced. Glandular hyperplasia with atypia is biologically and fundamentally different from cystic glandular hyperplasia and it is possible that the lesion called glandular hyperplasia with atypia is not a true hyperplasia but basically represents a neoplastic reaction. Therefore, glandular hyperplasia with atypia is generally considered a precancerous lesion.

Adenomatoid hyperplasia is rare but usually occurs focally in an otherwise normal endometrium and, therefore, there are no grounds for believing that it is related to estrogen stimulation.

2.4.5 Carcinoma in Situ of the Endometrium

By definition, carcinoma in situ of the endometrium is a noninvasive lesion and, therefore, a true carcinoma in situ of the endometrium is one in which the glands have undergone neoplastic change but in which there is no invasion of the endometrial stroma. Under the microscope, the glands can be seen to be increased in number and show all sorts of irregular and often bizarre convolutions. The stroma is obliterated because of the massive hyperplasia of the glandular elements (back-to-back crowding). The cells show a high degree of dedifferentiation, being polyhedral or rounded, closely packed, with heavily stained nuclei, loss of nuclear polarity, prominent nucleoli, and the formation of intraglandular bridges.

Carcinoma in situ of the endometrium is the most controversial lesion under discussion. Some authors do not use the term, preferring to group such cases with a typical hyperplasia (Novak and Rutledge 1948). Other authors may delineate some of these atypical hyperplastic patterns as carcinoma in situ of the endometrium (Hertig et al. 1949; Beutler et al. 1963; Vellions 1972). Welch and Scully (1977) stressed the cytologic features and limited extent of carcinoma in situ as important criteria for diagnosis. They pointed out that, if more than five or six glands are involved, the lesions are designated as carcinoma with the realization that invasion of the stroma is often impossible to distinguish from the crowding of noninvasive atypical glands. Gore and Hertig (1966) found that the more complex the pattern in hyperplasia the more likelihood of future invasive carcinoma. They stated that they have never observed carcinoma to arise from normal endometrium and that only rarely was cystic hyperplasia followed by carcinoma.

Atypical adenomatous hyperplasia of the endometrium is reported in the pathogenesis of endometrial carcinoma. It was documented by Gusberg and Kaplan (1963) in a study of 68 women with adenomatous hyperplasia, 12% of whom subsequently developed endometrial carcinoma. At the end of the 7th year of evaluation, the percentage of carcinoma in the hyperplasia group was statistically different from the percentage of matched controls ($P < 0.01$) without adenomatous hyperplasia.

The risk of developing endometrial carcinoma from precursor lesion reported in the literature is shown in Table 2.5. Wentz (1974) presented data on 115 patients with adenomatous hyperplasia, atypical hyperplasia, and carcinoma in situ using the criteria of Vellions (1972). Patients who had one of the three lesions on two curettage specimens at least 8 weeks apart were collected. Patients did not undergo hysterectomy and had not had hormonal therapy. A significant number of patients developed invasive endometrial carcinoma during the subsequent period of 2–8 years (Table 2.6).

Kurman et al. (1985) reported their long-term study on untreated endometrial hyperplasia in 170 patients. All of these patients were evaluated to correlate with

Table 2.5. Risk of developing endometrial carcinoma from a precursor lesion

Reference	Year	Precursor lesion	Eventual cancer (%)
Boronow	1976	Cystic hyperplasia	1–2
Koss	1980	Cystic hyperplasia	4
Chamblian and Taylor	1970	Adenomatous hyperplasia	14
Ferenczy	1978	Adenomatous hyperplasia	10

Table 2.6. Persistent Endometrial Hyperplasia: Premalignant Potential. Percentage of patients developing carcinoma within 2–8 years for three groups. (Adapted from Wentz 1974)

	No.	Percentage
Adenomatous hyperplasia	75	26.7
Atypical hyperplasia	22	81.8
Adenocarcinoma *in situ*	18	100.0

the histopathologic features with behavior. The mean follow-up period was 13.4 years. Cytologic and architectural alterations were analyzed separately in order to assess their respective roles in predicting the likelihood of progression to carcinoma. Proliferative lesions without cytologic atypia were classified as hyperplasia whereas those with cytologic atypia were classified as atypical hyperplasia. Subclassification of these two groups was based on the severity of architectural abnormalities. Hyperplasia and atypical hyperplasia displaying marked glandular complexity and crowding were designated complex hyperplasia (CH) and complex atypical hyperplasia (CAH), respectively. Lesser degrees of crowding were designated simple hyperplasia (SH) and simple atypical hyperplasia (SAH). Progression to carcinoma occurred in 1 (1%) of 93 patients with SH, 1 (3%) of 29 with CH, 1 (8%) of 13 with SAH, and 10 (29%) of 35 with CAH. The differences between the four subgroups suggest a trend but are not statistically significant. The findings provide a rationale for classifying endometrial hyperplasia primarily by cytologic atypia since this is the single and most useful criterion in predicting progression to carcinoma and secondarily by the existence of architectural abnormalities.

There is an accumulation of evidence to suggest that endometrial carcinoma is preceded by changes in the normal menstrual cycle. There is no proof that carcinoma may appear suddenly in an absolutely normal endometrium. There is evidence to suggest that the more complex the hyperplastic pattern the greater the likelihood of subsequent adenocarcinoma. The gradual morphologic transition from benign hyperplasia to neoplasia has been observed not only in sequential biopsy but on occasion in the same endometrium. The process of morphologic transition from normal endometrium to endometrial carcinoma is shown in Fig. 2.19.

2.4.6 Distinction Between Hyperplasia and Adenocarcinoma

Distinguishing between atypical adenomatous hyperplasia and well-differentiated adenocarcinoma may present certain problems. The difficulty is especially encountered in curettage material. The criteria suggested by Silverberg (1977), Tavassoli and Kraus (1978), Hendrickson and Kempson (1980), and Robertson (1981) indicate that:

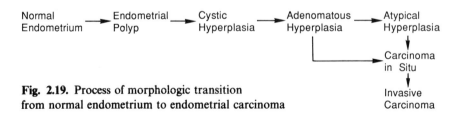

Fig. 2.19. Process of morphologic transition from normal endometrium to endometrial carcinoma

1. The glands are neoplastic rather than hyperplastic such as intraglandular bridging unassociated with intervening stroma, karyorrhectic debris within gland lumina, extensive interglandular proliferation and "daughter" gland formation, the loss of nuclear polarity, the presence of marked nuclear irregularity, the rounding of the nuclei, the prominence of the nuclei, the presence of pale eosinophilic cytoplasm, numerous mitotic figures or abnormal mitotic figures, the complete absence of stroma between glands, and the piling up of cells into sheets and masses.
2. Stromal invasion is of importance. This is best evaluated by observing the relationship between the glands and intervening stroma. The stroma may either disappear between the adjacent glands producing a back-to-back pattern or become fibrotic or even necrotic. Stromal accumulation of histiocytes may also be of malignant nature.

Based on clinical and pathologic analysis, Wu et al. (1982) suggested the following criteria for the differentiation of endometrial hyperplasia from endometrial carcinoma.

1. The morphologic pattern of glandular epithelium is an important factor. Severe atypical endometrial hyperplasia has the intact glandular epithelium but there is no intact glandular epithelium in endometrial carcinoma. Even the morphologic manifestation between endometrial hyperplasia and endometrial carcinoma is similar. If there is intact or flattened glandular epithelium, the diagnosis of endometrial carcinoma could be excluded. In addition, endometrial carcinoma is frequently associated with hemorrhage and necrosis.
2. Reaction to the progestins is useful for identification. Endometrial hyperplasia may rapidly react to therapy with one of the progestins at a comparatively lower dose. Cystic and adenomatous hyperplasia may undergo regression and the actively proliferating stroma may be converted to a decidual pattern by administration of synthetic progestational agents. In a short period, progestational agents will bring about endometrial atrophy and reversal of hyperplasia. For patients with endometrial carcinoma who have very definite medical contraindications to hysterectomy, only long-term constant administration of large doses of progestational agents may bring about reversal of endometrial carcinoma and recurrence might rapidly occur if administration of progestational agents stops.
3. Age is also an important factor for identification. All observations suggest that hyperplasia tends to occur at a younger age than carcinoma. Novak and Yui (1936) found that 4.8% of 804 patients with hyperplasia were over 55 years of age, while 59% of 104 patients with adenocarcinoma were over 55 years of age.

References

Aalders JG, Aderler V, Kolstad P (1984) Stage IV endometrial carcinoma: a clinical and histopathological study of 83 patients. Gynecol Oncol 17:75–84

Aguirre P, Scully RE, Wolfe JH, DaLellis RA (1983) Endometrial carcinoma with argyophil cells: a histochemical and immunohistochemical analysis. Presented at the International Academy of Pathology Meeting, Atlanta, March 1983

Albores-Saavedra J, Larraza O, Poucell S, Rodrigues-Martinez HA (1976) Carcinoma of the uterine cervix. Additional observations on a new tumor entity. Cancer 38:2328–2342

Albores-Saavedra J, Rodrigues-Martinez HA, Hernandez O (1979) Carcinoma tumor of the cervix. Pathol Annu 14:273–291

Atkin NB (1976) Cytogenetic aspects of malignant transformation. Exp Biol Med 6: 76–79

Baggish MD, Woodruff OD (1967) The occurrence of squamous epithelium in the endometrium. Obstet Gynecol Surv 22:69–115

Bamforth J (1956) Carcinoma of body of uterus and its relationship to endometrial hyperplasia: histological study. J Obstet Gynaecol Br Commonw 63:415–419

Bannatyne P, Russel P, Wills EJ (1983) Argyophilia and endometrial carcinoma. Int J Gynecol Pathol 2:235–254

Beck RP, Latour JPA (1963) Necropsy reports on 36 cases of endometrial carcinoma. Am J Obstet Gynecol 85:307–311

Benjamin I, Block RE (1977) Endometrial response to estrogen and progesterone therapy in patients with gonadal dysgenesis. Obstet Gynecol 50:136

Beutler HK, Dockerty MB, Randall LM (1963) Precancerous lesions of the endometrium. Am J Obstet Gynecol 86:433–443

Bibbo MC, Kapp DS, LiVolsi VA, Schwartz PE (1980) Squamous carcinoma of the endometrium with ultrastructural observations and review of the literature. Gynecol Oncol 10:217–223

Boronow RC (1976) Endometrial cancer and endometrial hyperplasia. In: Rutledge F et al. Gynecolgical Oncology 97–116 Wiley New York

Boutselis JG (1978) Endometrial carcinoma, prognostic factors and treatment. Surg Clin North Am 58:109

Broders AC (1925) The grading of carcinoma. Minn Med 8:726

Campbell PE, Barter RA (1961) The significance of atypical endometrial hyperplasia. J Obstet Gynecol Br Commonw 68:668–672

Chamblian DT, Taylor HB (1970) Endometrial hyperplasia in young women. Obstet Gynecol 36:659

Chen JL, Trost DC, Wilkinson EJ (1985) Endometrial papillary adenocarcinomas: two clinicopathological types. Int J Gynecol Pathol 4:279

Christopherson WM, Alberhasky RC, Connelly PJ (1982) Carcinoma of the endometrium I. A clinicopathologic study of clear-cell carcinoma and secretory carcinoma. Cancer 49:1511–1523

Connelly PJ, Alberhasky RC, Christopherson WM (1982) Carcinoma of the endometrium III, analysis of 865 cases of adenocarcinoma and adenoacanthoma. Obstet Gynecol 59:569–575

Coombes RC, Ward MK, Greenberg PB et al. (1976) Calcium metabolism in cancer. Studies using calcium isotopes and immunoassays for parathyroid hormone and calcitonin. Cancer 38:2111–2120

Cullen TH (1900) Cancer of the uterus. Saunders, Philadelphia

Dahle R (1956) Transtubal spread of tumor cells in carcinoma of the body of the uterus. Surg Gynecol Obstet 102:332–336

DiSaia PJ (1975) Cancer of the corpus. In: DiSaia PJ, Morrow CP (Eds.) Synopsis of gynecological oncology. New York, John Wiley & Sons 117

Ferenczy A, Richart RM (1974) Female reproductive system: dynamics of scan and transmission electron microscopy. Wiley, New York

Ferenczy A (1978) The histogenesis and cytodynamics of endometrial hyperplasia and neoplasia. In: Richardson GS, Machanglin DT (eds) Hormonal biology of endometrial cancer. International Union Against Cancer, Geneva

Feyrter F (1938) Über diffuse endokrinen epheliate Organe. Barth, Leipzig

FIGO (1970) Classification and staging of malignant tumors in the female pelvis, accepted by the General Assembly of FIGO in New York, Apr 12, 1970. Acta Obstet Gynecol Scand 50:1

Fluhmann CF (1928) Squamous epithelium in the endometrium in benign and malignant conditions. Surg Gynecol Obstet 48:309

Fox H (1983) Atypical hyperplasia and adenocarcinoma of the endometrium. In: Morrow CP et al. (eds) Recent clinical development in gynecologic oncology. Raven, New York, p 69–81

Frick HC, Munnell EW, Richart RM et al. (1973) Carcinoma of endometrium. Am J Obstet Gynecol 115:663–676

Gompel C, Silverberg SG (1985) The corpus uteri. In: Pathology in gynecology and obstetrics. Lippincott, Philadelphia 149–277

Gore H, Hertig AT (1962) Premalignant lesions of the endometrium. Clin Obstet Gynecol 5:1148–1165

Gore H, Hertig AT (1966) Carcinoma in situ of endometrium. Am J Obstet Gynecol 94:134–155

Granberg I, Gupta S, Joelsson I, Sprenger E (1974) Chromosome and nuclear DNA study of a uterine adenocarcinoma and its metastases. Acta Pathol Microbiol Scand (A) 82:1–6

Gray LA, Robertson RW Jr, Christopherson WA (1974) Atypical endometrial changes associated with carcinoma. Gynecol Oncol 2:93–100

Gusberg SB (1947) Precursors of corpus carcinoma: estrogens and adenomatous hyperplasia. Am J Obstet Gynecol 54:905–927

Gusberg SB, Kaplan AL (1963) Precursors of corpus cancer IV. Adenomatous hyperplasia as stage O carcinoma of the endometrium. Am J Obstet Gynecol 87:662–678

Haqqani MT, Fox H (1976) Adenosquamous carcinoma of the endometrium. Am J Clin Pathol 29:959–966

Hendrickson M, Kempson RL (1980) Surgical pathology of the uterine corpus. Saunders, Philadelphia

Hendrickson M, Ross J, Eifel P et al. (1982) Uterine papillary serous carcinoma: a highly malignant form of endometrial adenocarcinoma. Am J Surg Pathol 6:93–108

Henriksen E (1949) The lymphatic spread of carcinoma of the cervix and of the body of the uterus; a study of 420 necropsies. Am J Obstet Gynecol 58:924–940

Hertig AT, Sommers SC, Bengloff H (1949) Genesis of endometrial carcinoma, carcinoma in situ. Cancer 2:964–966

Hertig AT, Gore H (1960) Tumors of the female sex organs. Part 2; tumors of the vulva, vagina and uterus. Armed Forces Institute of Pathology, Washington DC

Homesley HD, Boronow RC, Lewis JL Jr (1977) Stage II endometrial adenocarcinoma: Memorial Hospital for Cancer, 1949–1965. Obstet Gynecol 49:604–608

Hopkin ID, Hawlow RA, Stevens PJ (1970) Squamous carcinoma of the body of the uterus. Br J Cancer 24:71–76

Inoue M, Veda G, Yamasaki M et al. (1984) Immunohistochemical demonstration of peptide hormones in endometrial carcinomas. Cancer 54:2127–2131

Jeffrey JF, Krepart GV, Lotocki RL (1986) Papillary serous adenocarcinoma of the endometrium. Obstet Gynecol 67:670–674

Jones HW (1975) Treatment of adenocarcinoma of the endometrium. Obstet Gynecol Surv 30:147–169

Katayama KP, Jones HW Jr (1967) Chromosomes of atypical (adenomatous) hyperplasia and carcinoma of the endometrium. Am J Obstet Gynecol 97:978–983

Kay S (1957) Clear cell carcinoma of the endometrium. Cancer 10:124–130

Kay S (1978) Squamous cell carcinoma of the endometrium. Am J Clin Pathol 61:264–269

Koss LG (1980) Recent advances in endometrial neoplasia. Acta Cytol 24:478

Kottmeier HL (1973) Annual report of the results of treatment in carcinoma of the uterus and vagina vol 15. International Federation of Gynecologic Oncology, Stockholm

Kumar NB (1984) Small cell carcinoma of the endometrium in a 23-year-old woman: light microscopic and ultrastructural study. Am J Clin Pathol 81:98–101

Kurman RJ, Scully RE (1976) Clear cell carcinoma of the endometrium: an analysis of 21 cases. Cancer 37:872–882

Kurman RJ, Kaminski PF, Norris HJ (1985) The behavior of endometrial hyperplasia: a long-term study of "untreated" hyperplasia in 170 patients. Cancer 56:403–412

Li SY (1988) Pathology. In: Li SY (ed) Endometrial carcinoma. People's Medical Publishing House, Beijing, p 26–57

Lutz MH, Underwood PB Jr, Kreutner A Jr, Miller MC (1978) Endometrial carcinoma; a new method of classification of therapeutic and prognostic significance. Gynecol Oncol 6:83–94

Melin JR, Wanner L, Schulz DM (1979) Primary squamous cell carcinoma of the endometrium. Obstet Gynecol 53:115–119

Morrow CP, DiSaia PJ, Townsend DE (1973) Current management of endometrial carcinoma. Obstet Gynecol 42:399–408

Mullins JD, Colonel LT, Hilliard GD (1981) Cervical carcinoid (argyophil cell carcinoma) associated with an endocervical adenocarcinoma: a light and ultrastructural study. Cancer 47:785–790

Ng ABP, Reagan JW, Storaasli JP et al. (1973) Mixed adenosquamous carcinoma of the endometrium. Am J Clin Pathol 59:765–790

Novak E, Yui E (1936) Relation of hyperplasia to adenocarcinoma of uterus. Am J Obstet Gynecol 32:674–781

Novak E, Rutledge F (1948) Atypical endometrial hyperplasia simulating adenocarcinoma. Am J Obstet Gynecol 55:46–61

Olson N, Twiggs L, Sibley R (1982) Small cell carcinoma of the endometrium: light microscopic and ultrastructural study of a case. Cancer 50:760–765

Paz RA, Frigerio B, Sundblad AS, Eusebi V (1985) Small cell (oat cell) carcinoma of the endometrium. Arch Pathol Lab Med 109:270–272

Pazdur R, Bonomi P, slayton R et al. (1981) Neuroendocrine carcinoma of the cervix: implications for staging and therapy. Gynecol Oncol 12:120–128

Pearse AGE (1969) The cytochemistry and cell structure of polypeptide hormone-producing cells of the APUD series and the embryological, physiological implications of the concept. J Histochem Cytochem 17:303–313

Pearse AGE (1974) The APUD cell concept of its implication in pathology. Pathol Annu 9:27–41

Plentl AA, Friedman AE (1971) Lymphatic system of the female genitalia. Saunders, Philadelphia, p 135

Poulsen HE, Taylor CW (1975) International classification of tumors no. 13. Histological typing of female genital tract tumors. WHO, Geneva

Prade M, Gadenne C, Duvillard P et al. (1982) Endometrial carcinoma with argyrophilic cells. Hum Pathol 13:870–871

Reagan JW, Fu YS (1981) Pathology of endometrial carcinoma. In: Coppleson M (ed) Gynecologic oncology. Churchill Livingstone, Edinbourgh, p 546–570

Richart RM (1973) Cervical intraepithelial neoplasia. Pathol Annu. 7–301

Robboy SJ, Bradley R (1979) Changing trends and prognostic features in endometrial cancer associated with exogenous estrogen therapy. Obstet Gynecol 54:269–277

Robertson WB (1981) The endometrium. Butterworths, London

Rosen SW, Weintraub BD (1974) Ectopic production of the isolated alpha subunit of the glycoprotein hormones. A quantitative marker in certain cases of cancer. N Engl J Med 290:1441–1447

Rosenwaks Z, Wentz AC, Jones GS et al. (1979) Endometrial pathology and estrogens. Obstet Gynecol 53:403–410

Ruffolo EH, Cavanagh D, Marsden DE (1983) Glandular intraepithelial neoplasia (CIN). A unifying concept of the precursors of endometrial carcinoma. Aust NZJ Obstet Gynecol 23:220–347

Rutledge FN (1974) The role of radical hysterectomy in adenocarcinoma of the endometrium. Gynecol Oncol 2:331

Salazar OM, Depapp EW, Bonfiglio Ta et al. (1977) Adenosquamous carcinoma of the endometrium. An entity with an inherent poor prognosis. Cancer 40:119–130

Sherman AI (1978) Precursors of endometrial cancer. Isr J Med Sci 14:370

Silverberg SG, Bolin MG, DeGiorgi LS (1972) Adenoacanthoma and mixed adenosquamous carcinoma of the endometrium: a clinicopathological study. Cancer 30:1307–1314

Silverberg SG, DeGiorgi LS (1973) Clear cell carcinoma of the endometrium. Clinical, pathologic and ultrastructural findings. Cancer 31:1127–1140

Silverberg SG (1977) Surgical pathology of the uterus. Wiley, New York

Stanley MA, Kirkland JW (1968) Cytogenetic studies of endometrial carcinoma. Am J Obstet Gynecol 102:1070–1079

Tateishi R, Wada A, Hayakawa K et al. (1975) Argyophil cell carcinoma (apudomas) of the uterine cervix: light and electron microscopic observations of 5 cases. Virchows Arch (Pathol Anat) 366:257–274

Tavassoli F, Kraus FT (1978) Endometrial lesions in uteri resected for atypical endometrial hyperplasia. Am J Clin Pathol 70:770–779

Taylor MC (1932) Endometrial hyperplasia and carcinoma of body of uterus. Am J Obstet Gynecol 23:309

Tohya T, Miyazaki K, Katabuchi H et al. (1986) Small cell carcinoma of the endometrium associated with adenosquamous carcinoma: a light and electron micriscopic study. Gynecol Oncol 25:363

Tseng PY, Jones HW Jr (1969) Chromosome constitution of carcinoma of the endometrium. Obstet Gynecol 33:741

Ueda G, Sato Y, Yamasaki M et al. (1978) Argyophil cell adenocarcinoma of the endometrium. Gynecol Oncol 6:467

Ueda G, Yamasaki M, Inoue M, Kurachi K (1979) A clinicopathologic study of endometrial carcinoma with argyophil cells. Gynecol Oncol 7:223

Vellions F (1972) Endometrial hyperplasia, precursors of endometrial carcinoma. Pathol Annu 201 7:201–227

Vellions L (1974) Endometrial hyperplasia and carcinoma in situ. Gynecol Oncol 2:152–161

Welch WR, Scully RE (1977) Precancerous lesions of the endometrium. Hum Pathol 8:503–512

Wentz WB (1974) Progestin therapy in endometrial hyperplasia. Gynecol Oncol 2:362–367

Wu BZ, Tang MY, Lang JH (1982) Endometrial carcinoma. In: Lin QZ (ed) Gynecologic oncology. People's Medical Publishing House, Beijing, p 85–104

3 Diagnosis of Endometrial Carcinoma

3.1 Clinical Manifestation

3.1.1 Age

Endometrial carcinoma is primarily a disease of postmenopausal women. The peak incidence between 55 and 59 years of age is later than for cervical cancer. Only 2%–5% of all cases are diagnosed before the age of 40 and there is a sharp drop in the incidence after 70 years of age. Only 20%–25% of cases occur in premenopausal women (Silverberg 1975; Mattingly 1985; Aalders et al. 1980; Malkasian et al. 1980).

In the 449 cases of endometrial carcinoma presented by Li (1988), the age ranged from 29 to 76 years. About 45% (202/449 cases) were found in the age group 50–59 years, 34.7% (156/449 cases) were in the premenopausal period, and only 10.2% of patients (45/449 cases) were under 40 years of age. Lang et al. (1978) showed a median age of 53.3 years in a group of 108 cases with endometrial carcinoma. The age range was from 26 to 71 years; 58.3% (63/108 cases) occurred in the 50- to 64-year age group, and only 12% (13/108 cases) were found before the age of 40 years.

3.1.2 Symptoms

3.1.2.1 Uterine Bleeding

Abnormal uterine bleeding is the cardinal symptom of endometrial carcinoma. Over 90% of endometrial carcinomas present initially as post-menopausal vaginal bleeding. In perimenopausal women, women with irregular menses associated with menometrorrhagia, or women still menstruating regularly after 50 years of age should be observed with suspicion. Approximately 87.1% of patients presented irregular vaginal bleeding from a group of 449 cases with endometrial carcinoma. While 85% of postmenopausal patients had vaginal hemorrhage (Li 1988), Lang et al. (1978) noted similar features in their review. About 96.3% of patients (104/108 cases) with endometrial carcinoma had abnormal vaginal bleeding and 95.5% (63/66 cases) of postmenopausal patients complained of uterine bleeding.

3.1.2.2 Vaginal Discharge

Approximately one-third of patients present a watery, pussy, or blood-stained discharge due to the cancerous exudation or a pyometra. This discharge may be associated with abnormal vaginal bleeding. About 55.9% (251/449 cases) were presented as abnormal vaginal discharge (Li 1988). Lang J-H et al. (1978) reported that 25% (27/108 cases) of patients had irregular vaginal discharge. In the postmenopausal woman, the presence of pyometra requires great care in excluding endometrial carcinoma.

3.1.2.3 Pain

A very small percentage of patients present with pain. Pain is rarely an early symptom. The suprapubic discomfort may be caused by a pyometra or uterine spasm. The patient with advanced disease may present continuous pain in the lower abdomen, lumbosacral, or lower extremital region. Approximately 24.5% (110/449 cases) of patients complained of lower abdominal or lumbosacral pain.

3.1.3 Pelvic Examination

Physical examination seldom reveals much in the early stage of endometrial carcinoma. On vaginal examination, the only positive findings may be a slightly enlarged uterus and slight bleeding from the cervical os. The uterus may, however, be enlarged due to fibrosis, adenomyosis, pyometra, or other tumors. The corresponding manifestation may be revealed if pelvic organs such as vagina, cervix, ovaries, fallopian tubes, parametrium, and peritoneum are involved in the carcinoma. In the 70 cases of endometrial carcinoma, 30% or 21 cases were found to be associated with leiomyomata after hysterectomy (Wu 1982). A pelvirectal examination is imperative to exclude extrauterine spread of the disease.

3.2 Diagnosis

It is not difficult to diagnose endometrial carcinoma if the patient has been fully investigated. The fractional curettage may be the simplest and most accurate diagnostic method.

3.2.1 Endometrial Sampling of the Uterine Cavity

Histologic examination of the endometrium has been the definitive diagnostic procedure. The fractional curettage should be performed and it should be used to collect the endocervical tissue and endometrial samples. The following are the indications for fractional curettage:

1. In the postmenopausal patient, abnormal vaginal bleeding or blood-stained discharge may cause great attention in excluding endometrial carcinoma using fractional curettage if cervical cancer and vaginitis have been excluded. Especially if the vaginal mucosa does not reveal atrophy in a patient long past the menopause, it is suggestive of a raised estrogen level and may point to a higher risk of endometrial carcinoma.
2. The patient with a history of excessive vaginal bleeding due to chronic anovulation and infertility is at risk of developing endometrial carcinoma and should be investigated by fractional curettage.
3. Repeated abnormal cytology and normal cervical biopsy should also indicate fractional curettage.
4. All patients with persistent symptoms despite normal cytology should be submitted to fractional curettage.

A sample of endometrium may usually be obtained by endometrial biopsy or endometrial curettage. Fractional curettage should always be performed if endometrial carcinoma is suspected. In addition to sounding and curettage of the uterine cavity including the lower segment of the uterus, it is imperative to obtain a separate endocervical curettage.

It is necessary to pay attention to the following when a fractional curettage is performed.

1. The patient should have no symptoms of infection such as normal temperature, normal blood count, and classification.
2. The vulva, vagina, and cervix are sterilized using the routine method. The strict sterilization operation procedure should be observed.
3. The endocervix is first curetted and the sample placed in a marked specimen pot of formalin; then the fundus and the anterior and posterior walls of the cavity are systematically curetted, placing each specimen separately into its own clearly marked pot of formalin. If the estrogen receptor or progesterone receptor is also measured, the amount of tissue should be at least 250 mg, which must be placed in another empty pot and kept cold and processed within hours, or frozen, preferably in liquid nitrogen, and stored at $-70°$C.
4. The cervix and internal os are completely dilated with Hegar's dilators, up to No. 5 if necessary because of a tight internal os. Gentle operation protects the patient from collapse because of uterine perforation and severe pain. If the patient appears to be in a state of collapse, the operation should be stopped immediately. The patient is placed in a supine position with her head lowered. Intravenous injection of 50–100 ml 50% glucose should be performed. Curettage may not be started again until the patient has recovered to a normal condition.
5. Even when the pathologic diagnosis is "inflammatory or necrotic tissue," endometrial carcinoma is also suspected, as it always coexists with infection, necrosis, or pyometra. Repeated fractional curettage should be considered.

3.2.2 Cytologic Examination

Unlike the examination of the uterine cervix, the cellular detection of endometrial lesions requires more care in sampling, optimal preservation of the specimen, more clinical information, great experience on the part of the microscopist, and a significant margin of error.

A pap smear is inadequate to screen for endometrial carcinoma; less than 50% of patients have abnormalities on the smear obtained from cervicovaginal cytologic samples.

Bibbo et al. (1979) reported that cervicovaginal cytologic sampling from the ectocervix and the posterior fornix or a combined ectocervical and endocervical smear will have a diagnostic accuracy of up to 60%. Ectocervical and endocervical smears in combination with a smear from the posterior fornix will have a diagnostic accuracy of up to 80% if they are correctly executed. Koss et al. (1982) reported that the routine ectocervical smear occasionally detects endometrial carcinoma in the asymptomatic patient. Therefore, it is not as reliable as a screening test. Until now none of these methods have had a diagnostic accuracy which can approach that of cytologic screening in cervical carcinoma.

Many mechanical devices have been developed for cytologic and tissue sampling of the endometrial cavity for outpatient examination. The detection rate for endometrial carcinoma is 85.7%–100% and that for premalignant endometrial lesions and failure rate is 3%–9% (Table 3.1).

The cytologic methods commonly used in obtaining cellular specimens for detecting endometrial carcinoma are as follows:

1. Posterior vaginal fornix aspiration: aspirating the exfoliate cells from the uterine cavity in the posterior vaginal pool
2. Endometrial aspiration smear: aspirating a cellular specimen from the endometrial cavity by gentle suction with a standard syringe (Cary 1943)

Table 3.1. Endometrial carcinoma: efficacy and accuracy of cytologic sampling methods

Series	Year	Method	Failure or unsatisfactory sample	Accuracy in diagnosing adenocarcinoma	Accuracy in diagnosing hyperplasia
Kawada and An-Foraker	1979	Isaacs cell sampler	3.0%	97.0%	58.2%
Barbaro et al.	1982	Negative pressure lavage	4.1%	90.9%	59.1%
Linden and Roger	1982	Mi-Mark Helix	6.2%–9%	85.7%	–
Pacifico et al.	1982	Jet-Wash	8.0%	100.0%	50.0%
Sedagal and Iversen	1983	Endoscan	6.0%	91.3%	40.0%

3. Endometrial brush technique: a soft brush is ensheathed in a tube during passage through the cervical canal and is pushed out of the tube once the internal os has been passed to sweep the endometrial surface (Ayre 1955).
4. Gravlee jet washer: The Gravlee jet washer is a double cannula with a seal to achieve negative pressure in the uterine cavity. It enables the physician to wash out and at the same time collect endometrial cells or tissue fragments. The collection sample should then be centrifuged (Gravlee 1969; White et al. 1973; Pacifico et al. 1982).

At present, cytologic examination remains an adjunct method for the diagnosis of endometrial carcinoma. The final diagnosis must be based on pathologic diagnosis of endometrium.

A combination of samples obtained by aspirating the cervical canal and intrauterine aspiration may provide an optimal screening procedure for women in the high-risk group of endometrial carcinoma.

3.2.3 Hysteroscopy

It has only been in the past 20 years that hysteroscopy, though founded by Pantaleoni in the nineteenth century, has been generally used. The application of hysteroscopy has become widespread because of the use of glass fiber bundles for light and image transmission and the advances in research on the medium used for dilatation of the uterine cavity and in lighting and photographic engineering. Hysteroscopy should confirm the intrauterine pathology. In current practice three different methodologies have gained acceptance:

1. Hysteroscopy or panoramic hysteroscope: By distending the uterine cavity with visualizing medium for dilatation of the uterine cavity, the uterine cavity can be observed.
2. Contact hysteroscope: The lining of the uterine cavity can be observed without the use of medium for dilatation of the uterine cavity. The endoscope is placed in immediate proximity to the epithelium for the evaluation of color contour, pattern, and consistency.
3. Microscopic hysteroscope: More accurate observation of the lesion is provided with variable magnification from 1 to 150 times.

3.2.3.1 Medium Used for Dilatation of the Uterine Cavity

There are two kinds of medium used for dilatation of the Uterine Cavity, either liquid or gas. The liquid medium includes saline, glucose, and dextran solution, CO_2 being the major source of gas medium. Though both liquid and gas medium have advantages and shortcomings, the liquid medium has been generally used for the reasons shown in Table 3.2 (Lindemann 1972; Lindemann 1974; Sugimoto 1975)

Table 3.2. Comparison of liquid and gas media in hysteroscopic examination

	Liquid media	Gas media
Media used for dilation	Saline glucose solution dextran solution	CO_2
Removal of blood and debris in uterus	Easy	Difficult
Detailed view of lesions	Easily obtained	Obscured by glare of reflected light
Leakage of media through tubes	Less	Much
Embolism of media	None	Possible

3.2.3.2 Technique

1. Preparation and sterilization for hysteroscopy is similar to that for dilatation and curettage.
2. The cervical canal is first examined without dilatation. The hysteroscope is applied in its outer sleeve to the external os of the uterus, which has been fixed by tenacula.
3. The cervical canal is dilated with Hegar's dilators up to No 7. Paracervical block anesthesia should be used if there is difficulty in dilation of the cervix.
4. The outer sleeve with the obturator may be inserted readily through the cervical canal just past the internal os. The obturator is removed and the hysteroscope is introduced in its place with saline rinsing. When the irrigating saline returns clear, the flow is stopped, and the uterine cavity may be dilated with medium and examined.
5. Observation begins near the internal os and then moves gradually upwards to the uterine fundus and the bilateral tubal cornua. Suspected lesions may be biopsied under visual control.

3.2.3.3 Findings of Endometrical Carcinoma

The hysteroscopic appearance of endometrial carcinoma is that of a pale blue or yellowish-gray tumor with a soft consistency. Endometrial carcinoma may be classified into four types: diffuse, circumscribed, exophytic, and endophytic. Most of the circumscribed types display exophytic growth, often accompanied by ulceration, necrosis, and infection. The hysteroscopic patterns of endometrial carcinoma may have the types shown in Figs. 3.1–3.4.

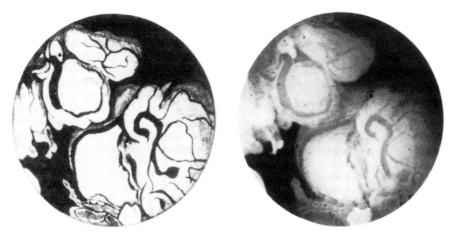

Fig. 3.1. Polypoid carcinoma of the endometrium. The almost smooth surface is crossed by engorged blood vessels. Histology showed tubular adenocarcinoma

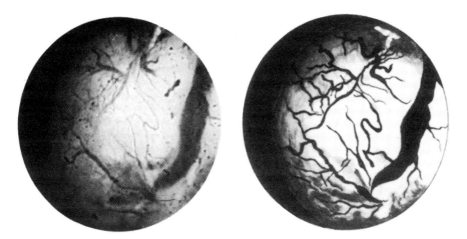

Fig. 3.2. Nodular carcinoma of the uterus with fairly smooth surface. The appearances resemble fibroid, but the blood vessels are thicker and more irregularly arranged

3.2.3.3.1 Polypoid Type

Endometrial carcinoma usually consists of several polypous protuberances with thin pedicles. The surface, light gray in colour, is rough and uneven, but it looks flat and velvety in some areas. The engorged vessels irregularly meander or zigzag on the surface. It should be differentiated from benign polyps, which may be rich in thin blood vessels and which are distributed in a regular fine network with no engorgement.

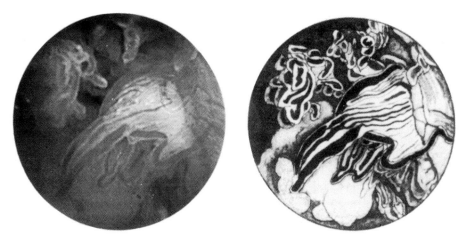

Fig. 3.3. Papillary carcinoma of the endometrium. The tumor is overgrown with long tentacle-like projections. Dilated vessels are characteristic

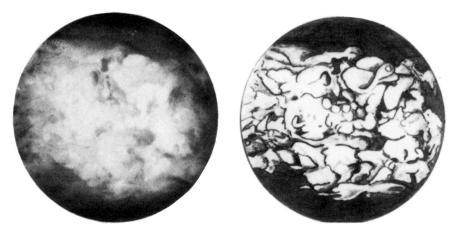

Fig. 3.4. Diffuse carcinoma of the endometrium. Necrotic tissue has sloughed, a finding peculiar to adenocarcinoma. Histology showed undifferentiated carcinoma

3.2.3.3.2 Nodular Type

Dilatation of blood vessels is more obvious, and they may form prominent varicosities which rise tortuously from the surface. Ulceration and infection also occur. It should be differentiated from submucous leiomyoma, which forms a hemispheric protrusion with a smooth surface. Subepithelial blood vessels are easily seen since the endometrium covering the nodule is stretched and thinned. These blood vessels are regularly arranged without engorgement. The peak incidence of leiomyoma is from the late reproductive age until just after the menopausal age.

3.2.3.3.3 Papillary Form

The surface of the endometrium is covered with numerous tentacle-like projections of cancerous tissues quivering in the rinsing saline. These tentacles, some long and others short, gather together and form a dendritic mass. Short tentacles resemble clusters of grapes, the long ones interlocking with each other like a ball of yarn. These tentacles are light pink in color as numerous cancer cells proliferate around the blood vessels.

3.2.3.3.4 Ulcerate Form

Necrosis and infection result in local ulceration, the surface of which is covered with pus or pieces of tissue and looks rough and fragile.

3.2.3.3.5 Diffuse Form

Cancer involves almost the entire uterine lining. The surface of the lesion is usually ragged and friable. The engorged vessels meander irregularly on the surface. Circumscribed polypoid change also occurred. Cancerous foci are usually not different from the surrounding endometrium as the cancerous foci do not rise so prominently. The formation of ulceration and increase in necrosis and pus on the surface make it difficult to estimate the original surface pattern and extension of tumor. If the necrotic tissue is washed away, the gray-yellowish, gray-reddish irregular, granular, and ragged cancerous foci will be discerned. The diffuse carcinoma should be differentiated from the benign polypoid hyperplasia of the endometrium and endometritis. The surface of polypoid hyperplasia of the endometrium is pink, smooth, and velvety. Diffuse carcinoma has a peculiar patch and variciform vascular pattern.

In general, the hysteroscopic characteristics of endometrial carcinoma are as follows:

1. As the growth becomes more vigorous and rapid, the tumor appears like a rough polyp, with nodular papilla or irregular projections.
2. The tumor surface looks gray-white, gray-yellowish, or dark-reddish because of hemorrhage, infection, and necrosis.
3. Marked varicosities and irregular dilatation of vessels are almost pathognomonic of endometrial carcinoma. These varicosities are dilated subepithelial blood vessels, mostly veins, which rise tortuously to the tumor surface.

3.2.3.4 Value of Hysteroscopy in the Diagnosis of Endometrial Carcinoma

Joelsson et al. (1971) suggested that hysteroscopy is very useful in the pre-treatment assessment of patients with endometrial carcinoma and may lead promptly to the most suitable treatment. Based on the histopathology of endometrial carcinoma, hysteroscopy may be used for the easy identification of intrauterine lesions. Hysteroscopy can determine the extent of the disease and whether the tumor is circumscribed or diffuse; it can observe the growth pattern and whether the tumor is exophytic or endophytic; and it can estimate whether the myometrium is invaded, and ascertain whether the cervix is involved. Sugimoto (1981) summarized the relationship between hysteroscopic findings and histopathologic patterns in 64 postmenopausal women with endometrial carcinoma. It is noted that many of the circumscribed carcinomas are well differentiated, while diffuse tumors are mostly poorly differentiated (Table 3.3). Endometrial carcinomas may be classified into two forms, diffuse and circumscribed, according to their hysteroscopic and histopathologic manifestation (Sugimoto 1981) (Fig. 3.5). Hysteroscopic studies suggest that the pattern of growth within the endometrial cavity reflects the aggresiveness of the tumor as measured by the depth of myometrial penetration (Tak et al. 1977). Anderson et al. (1980) reported that diffuse lesions and those with profuse endometrial growth were at greatest risk of myometrial penetration, so hysteroscopy may be used in predicting the presence of deep myometrial penetration.

Hysteroscopy allows for differentiation between overt involvement of cervical canal in endometrial carcinoma and endocervical adenocarcinoma (Baggish 1980; Bardot et al. 1980). At times hysteroscopy may also aid in the assessment of tumor regression following radiation therapy (Baggish and Bardot 1983). By performing hysteroscopy, it is possible to observe the endometrial changes, and more accurately directed endometrial biopsies can be obtained in young women undergoing hormonal therapy who have well-differentiated endometrial carcinoma and desire to have a baby.

Table 3.3. Endometrial carcinoma in postmenopausal women: relationship between hysteroscopic findings and histopathologic patterns. (Adapted from Sugimoto 1981)

Hysteroscopic patterns	Histopathologic patterns Differentiated (adenocarcinoma)			Undifferentiated
	Tubular	Adenomatous	Papillary	
Circumscribed type				
Polypoid type	4	2	–	–
Nodular type	7	7	2	–
Papillary type	–	–	24	–
Ulcerated type	1	5	6	3
Diffuse type	–	–	1	2

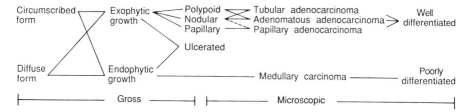

Fig. 3.5. Classification of endometrial carcinoma. (Adapted from Sugimoto 1981)

Hysteroscopy cannot replace endometrial biopsy in distinguishing between benign and malignant lesions, endometrial hyperplasia, and adenocarcinoma, or between the different grades and types of endometrial carcinoma (Sugimoto 1975). When the lesion encroaches on the internal carvical os, it may almost be impossible to distinguish between stage I and II disease. Du Toit (1985) reported understaged diagnosis in three cases (8.1%) and overstaged diagnosis in six cases (16.2%) in a series of 37 cases examined to distinguish between stage I and II disease.

It has been suggested that hysteroscopy could potentially cause dissemination of tumor cells (Valle Sciarra 1979). Baggish and Barbot (1983) also agreed with this opinion. Du Toit (1985) investigated this possibility by performing peritoneal cytology at laparotomy before hysterectomy for endometrial carcinoma. Peritoneal washing was performed for cytology at laparotomy before and after hysteroscopy. There was no proof that hysteroscopy spread malignant cells through the fallopian tubes. However, only 33 patients have been investigated and this issue remains unresolved.

3.2.4 Computerized Tomography

Computerized tomography (CT) can provide an excellent cross-sectional display of the pelvic organs and structures. There are two reasons for this. First, there is a large quantity of fat between the different organs and, secondly, the reproductive organs may not be affected by respiratory movement and intestinal peristalsis. The tumor location, size, shape, quality, and tumor invasion can be detected by CT scanning. In gynecological malignancy, the major roles of CT are in staging, monitoring response to treatment, and the detection of relapse.

3.2.4.1 Computerized Tomography Anatomy of Female Pelvic Organs

Computerized tomography can enhance the attenuation of X-rays, which permits the soft tissue structures to be distinguished from fat, air, and bone. Fat has a low density since it surrounds most pelvic organs and provides excellent contrast, which enables the various structures to be differentiated from each other.

1. Scans through the symphysis pubis show clearly the perineal muscles surrounding the urethra, vagina, and rectum. The ichiorectal fossae, bounded by the obturator internus and gluteus maximus muscles, are also obvious.
2. Scans passing just above the symphysis pubis show the bladder base, rectum, and vagina. The vaginal canal is outlined by air in the tampon.
3. Scanning above the vagina, the cervix can be identified as a smooth, rounded soft tissue structure 2–3 cm in diameter. The cervix and the body of the uterus cannot be reliably distinguished from each other, since there is no fat plane between them. On higher sections, the characteristic triangular shape of the uterus can be identified.
4. The ovaries are rarely identified on CT scans, presumably because there is little surrounding fat and they cannot be distinguished from adjacent vessels and nodes.
5. The ureters may be identified on several sections as they pass posteriorly to enter the bladder base.
6. The muscles of the pelvic side walls, such as the obturator internus and pyriformis, are clearly identified. The paired iliacus and psoas muscles are also recognizable on higher sections. The external and internal iliac arteries and veins and their accompanying lymph nodes lie close to the pelvic side walls but are not always identified as separate structures.

3.2.4.2 Method of Examination

1. The patient should take a suitable aperient on each of the preceding two nights.
2. Oral contrast medium (1% diatrizoate meglumine 250 ml) is given to delineate the small intestine and sigmoid colon, 12 h and 3 h before the examination, respectively. Some patients may also receive contrast enema to delineate the rectum and sigmoid colon.
3. Intravenous contrast medium (60% diatrizoate meglumine 30 ml) is used to show the bladder and ureters.
4. All married women are asked to insert a vaginal tampon to define the vaginal canal and uterine cervix.
5. The patient is asked to assume a supine position. Scanning is performed to take slices through the pelvis at 10-mm intervals, from the symphysis pubis to the level of the spina iliaca anterior superior. If the pelvic swelling lymph nodes are found, scanning is continued through the abdomen to the level of the nephric veins.

3.2.4.3 Computerized Tomographic Manifestation of Endometrial Carcinoma

1. Endometrial carcinoma is confined to the uterus, which may not be enlarged. Some tumors are isodense with the myometrium and, therefore, cannot be identified with CT.

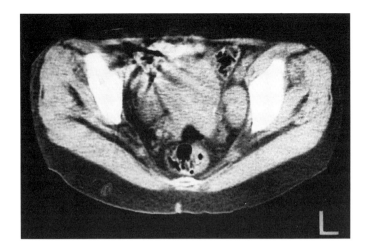

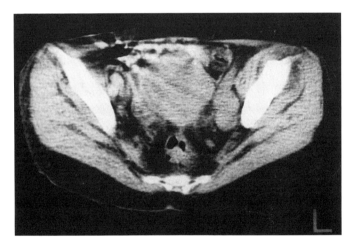

Figs. 3.6 (*above*), **3.7** (*below*). Computerized tomographic scans showing enlargement of the uterus and solid mass of the left parametrium in a 53-year-old woman with endometrial carcinoma. (Ye, Registry No. 372296, stage III, GII adenocarcinoma)

2. The tumor usually appears as an area of low density within the wall of the uterus. It enhances to a lesser degree than the normal myometrium following an injection of intravenous contrast medium.
3. The tumor may appear as a multilobular or triangle-shaped mass if it is invasive to adnexa. The tumor may involve the parametrial, paravaginal fat layer, bladder, rectum, and muscles of the pelvic side wall when it spreads widely.

3.2.4.3 Value of CT in Diagnosis of Endometrial Carcinoma

1. Computerized tomography can demonstrate extrauterine spread to the parametria, pelvic side walls, bladder, and rectum to help clinical staging.
2. The depth of myometrial invasion and the involvement of pelvic, abdominal lympth nodes should be seen and can serve as references for selecting an operation area and biopsy or resection of lymph nodes.
3. Residual and recurrent disease is seen either as a pelvic mass lying centrally, on the pelvic side wall, or as metastatic involvement of lympth nodes and the peritoneum. CT may help decide the most suitable form of treatment.

3.2.5 Magnetic Resonance Imaging

Magnetic resonance imaging (MRI) is a noninvasive method of mapping the internal structure of the body which completely avoids the use of ionizing radiation and appears to be unassociated with any significant hazards. It employs radio frequency (RF) radiation in the presence of a carefully controlled magnetic field in order to produce high-quality corss-sectional images of the body in any plane. It portrays the distribution density of hydrogen nuclei and parameters relating to their motion in cellular water and liquids. MRI has the advantage of being able to manipulate the contrast between different tissues in order to highlight pathologic changes by altering the pattern of RF pulse which is applied. As MR images of the pelvis are not degraded by respiratory motion because of the high inherent contrast between pelvic organs, fat, muscles, bowel gas, and urine in the bladder, high-quality images of the pelvis can be obtained.

3.2.5.1 Method of Examination

1. A suitable aperient should be taken on the preceding night as the rectum must be empty.
2. About 400–600 ml water is given to distend the bladder. The use of oral or parenteral contrast medium is not necessary.
3. All married women are asked to insert a vaginal tampon to define the vaginal canal and uterine cervix.
4. The patient is asked to lie on her back so that the pelvic cavity can be scanned.

3.2.5.2 Manifestation of Endometrial Carcinoma

1. The low-intensity line is normally seen at the endometrial-myometrial interface; the "junction zone" may be absent; there is often an irregular margin between the endometrium and myometrium. A widening of the endometrium may be revealed.

2. The signal intensity of the endometrium is inhomogeneous and abnormally high for the scanning sequence.
3. Endometrial carcinoma invading the myometrium and parametrium and metastazing to the lymph nodes would be clearly depicted on the MRI scan, causing thinning of the involved endometrium and asymmetrical enlargement of the myometrium, parauterine mass, and enlarged lympth nodes (Bies et al. 1984; Butler et al. 1984; Hricak et al. 1985; Thickman et al. 1984).

3.2.5.3 Value of MRI in the Diagnosis of Gynecologic Malignancies (Fig. 3.8)

Magnetic resonance imaging provides better delineation of the cervix from the uterine corpus than does CT. The superior contrast sensitivity of MRI provides

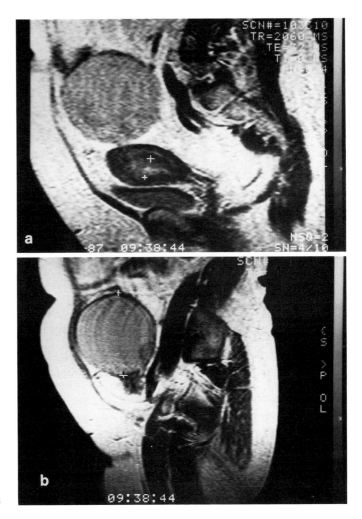

Fig. 3.8 a, b.
Legend see p. 74

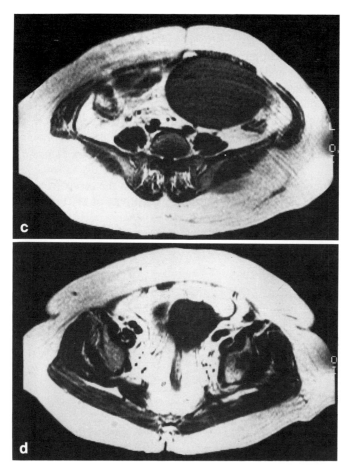

Fig. 3.8 a–d. Magnetic resonance imaging of endometrial carcinoma: 49-year-old woman (Yu, Registry No. 453139, endometrial carcinoma stage III). Cancer involves the whole interior of the uterus and is invasive to three-fourths of the myometrium. Pathologic diagnosis is endometrial adenosquamous carcinoma. Left ovarian metastatic adeno-squamous carcinoma. From sagittal T_2-weighted images and axial T_1-weighted images. **a,b** An enlarged uterus is identified with thickening of the endometrial layer, measuring approximately 2.1 cm, thinning of the myometrium in the anterior wall, and no delineation between the endometrial and myometrial layers in the posterior wall of the uterine corpus with increased signal intensity in the myometrial layer. **c, d** A left cystic structure with intact capsule and increased signal intensity on the region of the adnexa, representing a left cystic mass. The signal characteristics and morphology are consistent with that of an ovarian mass

separation of the endometrium not attainable with CT, and the extent of tumor invasion of the myometrium is more readily defined. Because of multiplanar imaging capacity, MRI is superior to CT in the depiction of the cephalocaudal extent of tumor. As the resolution of pelvic MRI is comparable to that of CT and as ionizing radiation and multiplanar scanning are not available, MRI may come to play a useful role in the assessment and staging of gynecologic malignancies.

3.2.6 Ultrasonographic Assessment of Endometrial Carcinoma

Diagnostic ultrasound has become an invaluable tool in the management of the patient with gynecologic cancer. It has been used in assessing tumor extent, following up the results of therapy and looking for tumor recurrence.
Sonographic diagnosis of endometrial carcinoma remains a difficult problem, despite the considerable experience gained over the past 10 years.

1. The normally homogeneous echo pattern of the uterus may be altered, or may even disappear. This change is not specific, because the heterogeneous echo pattern can be produced by endometriosis.
2. In more advanced disease with extensive replacement of the uterine parenchyma by tumor, the normal echo texture is replaced by an inhomogeneous pattern of high-level echoes interspersed among a background of relatively low-echo density. Areas of internal hemorrhage or hydrometra may be represented by irregular zones of fluid (Walsh et al. 1980; Requard et al. 1981).
3. In stage III disease, if the tumor extends into the adnexa or adjacent pelvic structures, a focal lobular mass extending out from the uterine body or an enlarged adnexal mass may present itself. It should be differentiated from the primary uterine tumor protruding from the uterine body, such as a leiomyoma.

3.2.7 Pelvic Lymphography

3.2.7.1 Indication

In patients with tumors of the genital organs, lymphography may be used to demonstrate lymph node metastases.

3.2.7.2 Contraindication

The examination is contraindicated in patients: (a) who have a known sensitivity to any of the agents used in the examination; (b) who have heart, liver, or kidney failure; or (c) who show severe exhaustion.

3.2.7.3 Technique

An attempt is made to cannulate a vessel in each foot or one side of the feet. After sterilization and anesthetization under aseptic conditions, 0.5 ml 1% methylene blue is injected into the two medial web spaces of the foot in order to make the lymphatics visible. Local anesthetic is injected and an incision is made over one of the lymphatic vessels (visible as thin blue lines stained with the blue dye). The vessel is cleared from the surrounding tissue. A No. 4 needle attached to a long polythene connection is used to puncture the lymphatic vessels. The syringe containing contrast medium is attached to the end of the polythene connection to start the injection. The contrast medium (Myodil 12–15 ml) is injected slowly and the speed is controlled at under 1 ml/5 min. After completion of the injection, a sequence of radiographs is taken. Anteroposterior views of the pelvis and abdomen and, if necessary, lateral and posterior oblique views should be taken immediately upon completion of the injection and 24 h afterwards.

3.2.7.4 Normal Manifestation

The inguinal, internal iliac, external iliac, and paraarotic lymph nodes are filled with contrast medium from the homolateral foot 24 h after the injection. The filling of lympth vessels up to the level of the second lumbar vertebra is deemed satisfactory. The contrast medium in the lymphatic vessels should be evacuated 24 h after completion of lymphography.

3.2.7.5 Abnormal Manifestation

1. For metastases, the most outstanding finding is the presence of a filling defect not transversed by lymphatic channels in a normal or enlarged lymph node.
2. If there is obstruction of lymphatic flow after 24 h of injection of contrast medium, numerous lymphographic pictures have been shown such as persistent contrast medium in lymph vessels, diameter of dilated vessels being more than 1 mm, extravasation of contrast medium, formation of collateral lymphatic flow, and dense accumulation of contrast medium in the periphery of the defect.
3. Nodal enlargement larger than 2.5 cm has pathologic significance.

3.2.7.6 Diagnostic Value in Endometrial Carcinoma

The direct relationship between pelvic, paraaortic lymph node metastases and pathologicosurgical staging, which is related to recurrence and prognosis, has been recognized. Lymphography can help determine whether lymph nodes are involved, therefore, it can be useful to make the treatment schedule. Musumeci et al. (1980) reported that in a group of 300 patients with endometrial carcinoma the incidence of metastases in recurrent patients was 47.5%, compared with 7.7% of patients without clinical evidence of disease. The prognostic significance of lymphography is evident enough to be able to carry out aggressive treatment in the positive cases (Table 3.4).

Table 3.4. Carcinoma of the endometrium: results of lymphography according to stage and presentation. (Adapted from Musumeci et al. 1980)

Stage or presentation	Cases (n)	Abnormal lymphography	
		(n)	(%)
I	115	9	7.8
II	28	4	14.3
III	29	11	37.9
IV	15	8	53.3
Total	187	32	17.1
Recurrence	61	29	47.5
Restaging, NED	52	4	7.7
Total	300	65	21.7

NED, no evidence of disease.

3.3 Differential Diagnosis

3.3.1 Differential Diagnosis of Endometrial Carcinoma

Endometrial carcinoma has no specific symptoms or physical signs and may associate with other kinds of tumors in the reproductive system and even pregnancy. Endometrial carcinoma should be distinguished from the following lesions:

1. Endometrial polyps and atypical hyperplasia
2. Uterine leiomyoma usually associated with endometrial carcinoma
3. Cervical cancer
4. Primary carcinoma of the fallopian tube
5. Endometritis and senile vaginitis

Differential diagnosis of the above lesions may be made with pelvic examination and pathologic examination, but if the cervix is invasive in endometrial carcinoma, it is sometimes very difficult to differentiate it from primary carcinoma of the cervical canal.

3.3.2 Association of Endometrial Carcinoma with Other Malignancies or Pregnancy

3.3.2.1 Coexistent Endometrial Carcinoma and Carcinoma of the Ovary

The coexistence of carcinoma in the ovary and endometrium is relatively uncommon but not rare. In general, it has been impossible to determine which of these tumors represent metastases from the endometrium or ovary or separate primary neoplasms, and gynecologists are unable to agree on the appropriate therapy. Kottmeier (1953), reporting the experience of a 30-year period at the Radiumhemmet in Sweden, noted simultaneous malignancies of the ovary and endometrium in 8.4% of the patients with endometrial carcinoma and 18.6% of the patients with ovarian carcinoma. Munnell and Taylor (1949) reported that in 28% of 190 (14.7%) patients with epithelial ovarian malignances the uterus was involved.

Previous investigators, in noting the simultaneous occurrence of ovarian and endometrial carcinoma, had difficulty in determining whether these neoplasms represented independent primary tumors or metastases. Matlock et al. (1982) suggested that the presence of different histologic subtypes in the two areas is a reliable criterion for differentiating primary from metastatic disease. Some investigators felt that, when the endometrial tumors were well differentiated, no more than 2 cm in size, and minimally invasive, it was best to consider them as separate primaries (Scully et al. 1966; Kurman and Craig 1972). The common findings of mixed epithelial neoplasms and the suggestion that epithelial tumors may be differentiated in different directions make the argument less compelling.

There has been uniform agreement that survival in cases of synchronous neoplasms of the ovary and endometrium is suprisingly good, and this relatively good survival has been used to argue that these tumors often represent separate primaries (Munnell and Taylor 1949; Kottmeier 1953; Dockerty 1954; Campbell et al. 1961; Schueller and Kirol 1966; Scully et al. 1966; Czernobilsky et al. 1972; Kurman and Craig 1972; Eifel et al. 1982; Matlock et al. 1982). To address the question of whether these neoplasms are synchronous separate primaries or carcinoma of the endometrium or ovaries with metastasis may provide useful information for determining therapeutically significant clinicopathologic groups.

3.3.2.2 Multiple Primary Gynecologic Malignancy

3.3.2.2.1 Definition

Two or more than two synchronous or metachronous (delayed) primary malignancies may be termed the multiple primary gynecologic malignancy.

3.3.2.2.2 Diagnosis Criteria

The diagnosis criteria of multiple primary tumors were defined by Warrens and Gates (1932): (a) each primary tumor must present its own definitive malignant pattern, (b) each primary tumor must be distinct, and (c) the probability of one tumor being a metastasis of the other must be excluded.

3.3.2.2.3 Incidence

Multiple malignant tumors were first described by Billroth in 1879. Since then many cases have been described and the incidence seems to be gradually increasing (Cahan 1977). Deligdisch and Szulman (1975) reported a 5.4% incidence of multiple carcinoma of the female organs and breasts. The reasons for the increasing incidence may be explained as follows:

1. Other carcinogenic factors such as irradiation, new chemotherapeutic agents, and new environmental contamination are considered as possible etiologic factors.
2. The increased longevity of cancer patients enables them to live long enough to develop multiple primary tumors.
3. The currently improved clinical awareness increases the diagnostic rate.

Cancer of the breast, ovary, and colon seems to occur more frequently in endometrial carcinoma. Schwartz et al. (1985) reported an epidemiologic study of multiple primary malignant tumors in 1007 patients with endometrial carcinoma in Israel between the years 1969 and 1975. A total of 104 (10.3%) patients with endometrial carcinoma had multiple primary malignancy. Four different sites such as the breast, ovary, cervix, and colon had a statistically significant, higher than expected incidence of secondary primary carcinoma. Various publications showed multiple primary cancers involving the breast, ovary, and large intestine to occur more frequently in patients with endometrial carcinoma than would be expected by chance (Moertel et al. 1961; Bailar 1963; Cook 1966; MacMahon and Austin 1969; Schoenberg et al. 1969; Vongtama et al. 1970; Schottenfeld and Berg 1971; Schoenberg 1977). Details on the number of multiple primary malignancies at different anatomic sites from three reports are shown in Table 3.5.

3.3.2.2.4 Etiology

It seems most likely that no one etiologic factor is responsible for the associated multiple primary tumors and their development is a function of multiple carcinogenic factors acting on possibly different and genetically predisposed hosts. If the multiple primary tumors appear either simultaneously or after successful treatment of an initial primary endometrial carcinoma, a possible associated etiology should be considered. If the interval between the identification of the endometrial carcinoma and the second primary tumors is considerable, the carcinogenic effects of irradiation, new chemotherapeutic agents, and environmental carcinogenic forces should be considered.

Table 3.5. Association of other tumors with endometrial carcinoma

	Malkasian et al. 1980	Axelrod et al. 1984	Li 1988
Endometrium	577	217	449
Cervix	0	2	10
Vulva	0	2	0
Vagina	0	2	0
Ovary, fallopian tubes	14	9	1
Breast	32	2	5
Colon, rectum, anus, sigmoid	25	2	5
Leukemia	3	1	1
Stomach	0	0	1
Liver	0	0	1
Esophagus	0	0	2
Appendix	2	0	1
Lymphoma	3	0	3
Pituitary adenoma	1	0	0
Thyroid	4	0	0
Lung	1	0	0
Bladder	2	0	0
Kidney	1	0	0
Liposarcoma	1	0	0
Fibrosarcoma	1	0	0
Melanoma	1	0	0
Squamous cell[a]	1	0	0
Total	92	20	30
Percentage	15.9	9.2	6.7

[a] Primary site unknown.

3.3.2.2.5 Prognosis

The prognosis of patients with second primary cancer depends on the type and malignancy of the second primary cancer. It is important to become aware of the possible occurrence of second primary tumor in patients with endometrial carcinoma. Knowing the specific sites at which the second cancer might appear may help in the early diagnosis of the cancer and thus improve the prognosis. Triple primary gynecologic malignancy is very rare since Day reported the first case in 1958, as only two cases had been described up to 1984. Gaulayev et al. (1984) reported a 71-year-old woman complaining of postmenopausal vaginal bleeding. Total abdominal hysterectomy and bilateral salpingo-oophorectomy and left mastectomy were performed. The diagnosis was endometrial adenocarcinoma, squamous cell carcinoma of the cervix, and infiltrating duct carcinoma of the breast.

3.3.2.3 Coexistent Immature Teratoma of the Uterus and Endometrial Adenocarcinoma Complicated by Gliomatosis Peritonei

In 1985, Ansah-Boateng et al. reported that a 37-year-old nulliparous woman complaining of severe vaginal bleeding underwent total hysterectomy with bilateral wedge resection of the ovaries. The pathologic diagnosis was immature teratoma of the uterus and well-differentiated endometrial adenocarcinoma. Mature glial implants were present on the ovaries and throughout the omentum. She was given a short course of pelvic radiotherapy. Two years later, she remains very well with no evidence of recurrence. Primary teratoma of the uterus is rare (Nicholson 1956; Pyrah and Redman 1968; Mold, 1969). The results of analysis of this disease are as follows:

1. Extragonadal teratomata may arise in sites to which germ cells normally migrate in the early embryonic life (Fox and Langley 1976).
2. Uterine teratoma represents residual fetal tissues remaining in the uterus for a number of years following a missed abortion or an undelivered papyraceous twin (Tyagi et al. 1979).
3. Uterine teratomata arise either from a germ cell which has gone astray during embryogenesis or from a germ cell which was primarily intraovarian but which has passed into the uterus and become arrested. The associated endometrial adenocarcinoma in this patient was the most interesting incidental finding although its relationship to the teratoma remains obscure. The presence of well-differentiated peritoneal implants is associated with a good prognosis. This apparently unique uterine teratoma with immature neuroepithelium has behaved as would have been expected of an equivalent ovarian tumor.

3.3.2.4 Adenocarcinoma of the Endometrium Associated with Intrauterine Pregnancy

The association of endometrial carcinoma with pregnancy is an extremely rare phenomenon. Since Schumann (1927) reported a patient having endometrial carcinoma coexistent with intrauterine pregnancy, only seven acceptable cases had been found in the literature until 1984, as summarized in Table 3.6. The apparent rarity of the association of endometrial carcinoma with pregnancy may be related to the following factors:

1. Endometrial carcinoma generally occurs in the postmenopausal period and only 3%–8% occur in women below 40 years of age (Kempson and Pokorny 1968; Creasman and Weed 1981).
2. The young patients prone to endometrial carcinoma frequently have an ovulatory disorder such as polycystic ovary syndrome and are, therefore, suspected of being less fertile.

Pregnancy would mask or lead to a misinterpretation of the principal signs and symptoms of endometrial carcinoma, so the possibility of endometrial carcinoma should be considered during pregnancy with irregular vaginal bleedings.

3.3.3 Rare Cases of Endometrial Carcinoma

1. Morris et al. (1985) reported three unusual patients who first manifested malignant ascites without vaginal bleeding and were considered to have ovarian cancer preoperatively. It should be noted that all were in their 8th decade, above the mean age of endometrial carcinoma. Laparotomy revealed gross omental tumor and normal ovaries. The endometrial carcinomas were grossly undetected and were uniformly noninvasive of the myometrium. One should consider endometrial carcinoma in the differential diagnosis of any postmenopausal patients with ascites even in the absence of vaginal bleeding.
2. Beller et al. (1984) presented a case of stage IV endometrial carcinoma having spontaneous regression of cancer. A 56-year-old white female was diagnosed as having stage IV endometrial carcinoma in exploratory laparotomy. A total abdominal hysterectomy and bilateral salpingo-oophorectomy was performed to avoid further vaginal bleeding. Postoperatively, progestational agents were taken for 3 weeks and local radiation therapy was given using an applicator for a total surface dose of 60 Gy. She was survived for 18 years without evidence of disease. A review of spontaneous regression of gynecologic cancers reveals that most reported cases were in situ carcinoma of the cervix (Conference on spontaneous regression of cancer 1966; Richard and Barron 1969; Ayre and Narvaez 1973). Although Everson and Cole (1966) reported seven cases of epithelial ovarian cancer and two cases of endometrial carcinoma, none demonstrated long-term survival. Although spontaneous regression does occur, the characteristics of such a phenomenon are still unknown.
3. Alenghat and Talerman (1982) reviewed a case of adenocarcinoma of the vermiform appendix manifesting itself as an endometrial carcinoma. A 78-year-old white female complained of postmenopausal bleeding and was initially considered to have endometrial carcinoma. An exploratory laparotomy revealed that the appendiceal tumor was associated with a diffuse metastatic process affecting the uterus, fallopian tubes, ovaries, and peritoneal cavity.

Although metastatic carcinoma to the uterus is uncommon, when evaluating an endometrial curettage containing neoplastic tissue, the possibility of metastatic carcinoma should always be considered. The neoplasms most frequently associated with metastases to the uterus are carcinomas of the breast, gastrointestinal tract, and kidney, and malignant melanoma.

In a period of 2 years, besides this case, a patient with carcinoma of the breast and a patient with carcinoma of the colon complained of abnormal vaginal bleeding and uterine metastases. In the case of metastatic carcinoma of the breast, the uterus, ovaries, and fallopian tubes were nearly completely replaced by tumor deposits without producing enlargement of any of the organs. Endometrial curettage in each case demonstrated an invasive adenocarcinoma with appearances which were not considered typical of primary endometrial origin. It is, therefore, considered that, in cases where the tumor seen in uterine curettings does not show typical appearances of endometrial carcinoma, careful investigation to exclude its possible extrauterine origin is mandatory.

4. Savage et al. (1987) presented a 70-year-old female with endometrial adenocarcinoma, focally differentiating to choriocarcinoma and metastasizing to the liver, brain, and lung as pure choriocarcinoma.

Choriocarcinoma arising from nonovarian, nongestational, and nonteratomatous settings has appeared in various organs (McKechnie and Fechner 1971; Civantos and Rywlin 1972; Park and Reid 1980; Saigo and Rosen 1981; Saigo et al. 1981; Knapp et al. 1982; Obe et al. 1983). Gastric choriocarcinoma seems to be the most common. Several cases of this carcinoma arising in the breast, colon, liver, esophagus, small bowel, prostate, bladder, lung, and nose have been reported (Saigo et al. 1981; Wurzel and Brooks 1981). Primary gynecologic choriocarcinoma arising in the uterus, vagina, or fallopian tube without germ cell tumors or preceding gestation have been described (Maizels 1940; White 1955; Latrop et al. 1978; Carenza et al. 1980; Lawrence 1984). This case of primary choriocarcinoma of the endometrium unrelated to gestation appeared first in the literature. Lawrence (1984) experienced a case of choriocarcinoma coexisting with adenosquamous carcinoma of the uterus. It is known that nearly half of the patients suffering from chorinocarcinomas of the uterus do not have a hisoty of hydatidiform mole. White (1955) reported that choriocarcinoma has not been infrequently observed in postmenopausal women. Choriocarcinoma of the uterus, particularly in postmenopausal women, may originate from the endometrium as adenocarcinoma and differentiate as trophoblasts without fertilized ova as precursors.

5. Zarian et al. (1983) described a case of endometrial adenocarcinoma metastasizing to the esophagus. A 71-year-old patient underwent a total abdominal hysterectomy and bilateral salpingo-oophorectomy as well as pelvic radiation therapy for stage I grade 2 endometrial adenocarcinoma 3 years previously. Pathologic evaluation revealed 50% myometrial penetration and lymphatic involvement. Six months later, a follow-up esophagram revealed a short segment of concentric narrowing in the mid-esophagus with intact overlying mucosa. Endosopic biopsy of the region was negative. Three months after this biopsy was performed, the patient experienced dysphagia A repeated esophagram revealed a longer, constricting lesion with ulceration in the area of the previously noted narrowing. Endoscopic biopsy of the lesion at this time revealed adenocarcinoma identical histologically to the original endometrial carcinoma. Pathophysiologically, it is believed that secondary involvement of the esophagus occurs by three mechanisms: direct extension, involvement by mediastinal lymph nodes containing tumor, and hematogenous spread (Fisher 1976). Since mediastinal lymph node enlargement was

Table 3.6. Summary of the reported cases with endometrial cacrcinoma in pregnancy

Series	Year	Age (years)	Parity	Symptoms	Gestational age (weeks)
Schumann	1927	43	10	Vaginal bleeding	10–12
Westman	1934	40	3	Vaginal bleeding with cramping	Not stated
Wallingford	1934	35	5	Amenorrhea	16
Wall and Lucci	1953	36	2	Postcoital bleeding, menorrhagia	28
Marinaccio and Mazzarella	1967	28	2	Intermenstrual spotting	Term
Karlen et al.	1972	21	2	Hypermenorrhea and dysmenorrhea	6–8
Sandstrom et al.	1978	37	0	Intermenstrual spotting	
Suzuki et al.	1984	30	1	Vaginal bleeding with cramping after amenorrhea	7

NED, no evidence of disease; TAH, total abdominal hysterectomy; BSO, bilateral

not observed with computerized tomography in this case, the metastatic endometrial adenocarcinoma to the esophagus is presumed to have spread by the hematogenous route.

3.4 Clinical Staging

Once the diagnosis of endometrial carcinoma is established, the stage of the disease has to be ascertained in order to decide the best therapeutic approach, compare the treatment results, and estimate the prognosis. The UICC staging for endometrial carcinoma was presented in 1968 but has not been used very often. The International Federation's (FIGO) classification for endometrial carcinoma has been in use since 1 January 1971 (Table 3.7) (FIGO 1977). Patients with stage I account for about 75%, while the remaining stages account for 25%. Currently, stage II requires the presence of carcinoma that involves, is contiguous to, or is directly beneath the endocervical glands. The problem inherent in the use of

Detection of carcinoma	Pathology	Treatment and prognosis
Endometrial biopsy, pregnancy was noted in the resected uterus	Adenocarcinoma	TAH, BSO; NED 20 months posthysterectomy
At D and C for spontaneous abortion	Adenocarcinoma	TAH, BSO; no residual tumor in the resected uterus
At D and C after spontaneous abortion	Adenocarcinoma polypoid, superficial, myometrial invasion	NED over 10 years after TAH, BSO
Biopsy of polypoid tissue from cervical os during pregnancy	Adenoacanthoma, diffuse involvement	Live infant by CS, died of recurrence 3 years after radium, TAH, BSO
Currettage twice before pregnancy	Adenoacanthoma, diffuse, well differentiated	Refused treatment: normal delivery 14 months after diagnosis, NED at 10 years
Curettage before pregnancy was noted	Adenoacanthoma focal non-invasive	NED 6 years, posthysterectomy
At D and C for therapeutic abortion	Adenoacanthoma, well differentiated, focal noninvasive	NED $2\frac{1}{2}$ years after TAH, BSO
At D and C for inevitable abortion	Adenocarcinoma, moderately differentiated, myometrial invasion	NED 5 years after TAH, BSO, external irradiation to pelvis

salpingo-oppohorectomy, CS, cesarean section.

fractional curettage and the possibility of overstaging of disease has been demonstrated (Surwit et al. 1978). The false-positive rate was 56.1% (37/66 cases). A total of 66 patients were diagnosed as having clinical stage II (Li 1988 Wallin et al. (1984) reported the false-positive rate to be 39% (18/46 cases) in the Mayo Clinic. The reasons for the false-positive results of clinical stage II endometrial carcinoma may include:

1. The tumor was polypoid in nature and originated from the upper or lower uterine segment.
2. A curettage sample failed to show endocervical glandular involvement.
3. Cancer was consistent with the development of a false canal in curettage and subsequent seeding of the passage with carcinoma.

The cervix is involved macroscopically or microscopically. If the cervix is involved macroscopically, it may be enlarged grossly, which may give it a nodular appearance. The outgrowth of cancer nodules from the cervical canal is of bulkier appearance. The naked involvement of the cervix would, therefore, predict a worsening of the prognosis. Among the 7561 women in 17 individual studies cited by Rutledge, 881 or 11.6% presented with cervical involvement (clinical stage II endometrial carcinoma) (Rutledge 1974). Li (1988) reported the incidence of cervical involvement in 418 patients with endometrial carcinoma to be 5.8%.

In stage III carcinoma of the endometrium, the tumor extends outside the uterus, but not beyond the true pelvis. There must be no involvement in the bladder or rectum. The involvement in the parametrium, vagina, or parametrium and vagina should be diagnosed as stage III, but the tumor spread to the parametrium is only clinically detectable.

In stage IV carcinoma of the endometrium, the tumor has extended outside the true pelvis or has obviously involved the mucosa of the bladder and/or rectum. Involvement in distant organs may occur in the following order: lung, multiple sites, upper abdomen, bone, brain, liver, and lymph nodes (Aalders et al. 1984). The clinical staging of endometrial carcinoma has certain inherent short-comings, the most important being that it depends on a clinical evaluation.

1. In stage I disease, the FIGO staging does not allow for the depth of myometrial invasion or for the distance of the tumor from the internal cervix os. These factors may severely influence the eventual prognosis. The depth of myometrial invasion may be determined on the basis of pathologic examination only. It has been difficult to assess accurately the myometrial invasion in patients who have received preoperative irradiation due to the interval between irradiation and operation.
2. In stage I disease, the size of the uterus must be accurately assessed to make possible differentiation between stage IA and IB diseases. The enlarged uterus caused by endometrial carcinoma may infer a worse prognosis (Jones 1975). Concomitant benign lesions of the uterus like leiomyoma or adenomyosis may, however, contribute to the enlargement in size of the uterus, and in such cases the uterine enlargement may not necessarily infer a worse prognosis.
3. In stage II disease, the false-positive rate of cervical involvement may be up to 30% due to the lack of a standardized procedure for the establishment of cervical involvement. Fractional curettage may be misleading unless the cancer is identified in continuity with recognizable cervical tissue.
4. In stage III disease, if the parametrial involvement is clinically detectable, most of the patients are technically inoperable and it is hardly surprising that the prognosis for these patients is poor.

Lewis et al. (1970) reported that the discrepancy between FIGO staging and surgicopathologic staging was 12%. Creasman et al. (1976) reported the results of a prospective study by the Gynecologic Oncology Group (GOG) in America, in which 23 patients (11.2%) of a group of 206 patients with stage I disease had one or more pelvic nodes involved. A definite correlation between lymph node involvement and the size of the uterus, the grade of the tumor, and the depth of myometrial invasion was observed.

Table 3.7. Endometrial carcinoma: FIGO staging classification (January 1971)

Stage O	Carcinoma in situ. Histologic findings of suspected malignancy (cases of stage O should not be included in any therapeutic statistics)
Stage I	The carcinoma is confined to the corpus
	Stage IA: the length of the uterine cavity is 8 cm or less
	Stage IB: the length of the uterine cavity is > 8 cm
	Stage I cases should be subgrouped with regard to the histologic type of adenocarcinoma as follows:
	G_1: highly differentiated adenomatous carcinoma
	G_2: differentiated adenomatous carcinoma with partly solid areas
	G_3: predominantly solid or entirely undifferentiated carcinomas
Stage II	The carcinoma has involved the corpus and cervix
Stage III	The carcinoma has extended outside the uterus but not outside the true pelvis
Stage IV	The carcinoma has extended outside the true pelvis or has obviously involved the mucosa of the bladder or rectum. A bullous edema, as such, does not permit assignment of a case to stage IV

These shortcomings in the clinical staging have a severe and negative impact on the prognosis of patients with endometrial carcinoma. Histologic grading, cell type, depth of myometrial invasion, and patient age may influence the prognosis especially in stage I disease (Berman et al. 1980). The combination of FIGO staging and surgicopathologic staging would be a reasonable method for estimating the area of cancer involvement and selecting the best therapy schedule.

References

Aalders JG, Abeler V, Kolstad P et al. (1980) Post-operative external irradiation and prognostic parameters in stage I endometrial carcinoma: clinical and histopathologic study of 540 patients. Obstet Gynecol 56:419–427

Aalders JG, Abeler V, Kolstad P (1984) Recurrent adenocarcinoma of the endometrium: a clinical and histopathological study of 379 patients. Gynecol Oncol 17:85–103

Alenghat E, Talerman A (1982) Case report adenocarcinoma of the vermiform appendix presenting as a uterine tumor. Gynecol Oncol 13:265–268

Ansah-Boateng Y, Wells M, Poole DR (1985) Coexistent immature teratoma of the uterus and endometrial adenocarcinoma complicated by gliomatosis peritonei. Gynecol Oncol 21:106–110

Anderson B, Louis F, Watring WG, Edinger DD Jr (1980) Growth patterns in endometrial carcinoma. Gynecol Oncol 10:134–145

Axelrod JH, Fruchter R, Boyce JG (1984) Multiple primaries among gynecologic malignancies. Gynecol Oncol 18:359–372

Ayre JE (1955) Rotating endometrial brush: new technic for the diagnosis of fundal carcinoma. Obstet Gynecol 5:137

Ayre SE, Narvaez R (1973) Carcinoma in situ: behavior patterns and cytoimmunology. Oncology 27:294–304

Baggish MS (1980) Evaluation and staging of endometrial and endocervical adenocarcinoma by contact hysteroscopy. Gynecol Oncol 9:182–192

Baggish MS, Barbot J (1983) Contact hysteroscopy. Clin Obstet Gynaecol 26:219–241

Bailar JG III (1963) The incidence of independent tumors among uterine cancer patients. Cancer 16:842–853

Barbaro CA, Fortune DW, Bodey AS et al. (1982) Uterine-lavage in the diagnosis of endometrial malignancy and its precursors. Acta Cytol 26:135–140

Bardot J, Parent B, Dubuisson J (1980) Contact hysteroscopy: another method of endoscopic examination of the uterine cavity. Am J Obstet Gynecol 136:721–726

Beller V, Beckman EM, Twombly GH (1984) Spontaneous regression of advanced endometrial carcinoma. Gynecol Oncol 17:381–385

Berman ML, Barlow SC, Lagasse LD et al. (1980) Prognosis and treatment of endometrial cancer. Am J Obstet Gynecol 136:679–688

Bibbo M, Reale FR, Reale JC et al. (1979) Assessment of three sampling technics to detect endometrial cancer and its precursors. Acta Cytol 23:353–359

Bies JR, Ellis JH, Kopecky KK et al. (1984) Assessment of primary gynecologic malignancies of 0.15T resistive MRI with CT. Am J Roentgenol 143:–1249

Billroth T (1879) Chirurgische Klinik in Wien 1871–1876 mit einem Gesamt-Bericht über die chirurgischen Kliniken in Zürich und Wien während der Jahre 1860-1876 Erfahrungen auf dem Gebiete der praktischen Chirurgie. Hirschwald, Berlin p258

Butler H, Bryan PJ, Lipuma Jr et al. (1984) Magnetic resonance imaging of the abnormal female pelvis. Am J Roentgenol 143:1259–1266

Cahan WG (1977) International workshop on multiple primary cancer. Introductory remarks. Cancer 40:1785

Campbell JS, Magner D, Fournier P (1961) Adenoacanthomas of ovary and uterus occurring as coexistent or sequential primary neoplasms. Cancer 14:817–826

Carenza L, DiGregorio R, Mocci C et al. (1980) Ectopic human chorionic gonadotropin: gynecologic tumors and non-malignant conditions. Gynecol Oncol 10:32–38

Cary WHA (1943) A method of obtaining endometrial smear for study of their cellular content. Am J Obstet Gynecol 46:422–424

Civantos F, Rywlin AD (1972) Carcinomas with trophoblastic differentiation and secretion of chorionic gonadotropins. Cancer 29:789–797

Conference on spontaneous regression of cancer (1966) NCI Monogr:44

Cook GBA (1966) A comparison of single and multiple primary cancers. Cancer 19:959–966

Creasman WT, Boronow RC, Morrow CP et al. (1976) Adenocarcinoma of the endometrium: its metastatic, lymph node potential. Gynecol Oncol 4:239–243

Creasman WT, Weed JC Jr (1981) Carcinoma of endometrium (FIGO Stage I and II): clinical features and management. In: Coppleson M (ed) Gynecologic oncology: fundamental principles and clinical practice. Churchill Livingstone Edinbourgh, 571–577

Czernobilsky B, Silverman BB, Mikuta JJ (1972) Endometrial carcinoma of the ovary. Cancer 26: 1142–1152

Day JC (1958) The second primary malignant tumor in gynecology: review of the literature and series presentation. Am J Obstet Gynecol 75:976–982

Deligdisch L, Szulman EE (1975) Multiple and multifocal carcinomas in female genital organs and breast. Gynecol Oncol 3:181–190

Dockerty MB (1954) Primary and secondary ovarian adenocanthoma. Surg Gynecol Obstet 99: 392

Du Toit JP (1985) Carcinoma of the uterine body. In: Shepherd JH, Monaghan JM (eds) Clinical gynaecological oncology. Blackwell, Oxford, 97–132

Eifel P, Hendrickson M, Ross J et al. (1982) Simultaneous presentation of carcinoma involving the ovary and uterine corpus. Cancer 50:163–170

Everson TC, Cole WH (1966) Spontaneous regression of cancer. Saunders, Philadelphia

FIGO (1970) Classification and staging of malignant tumors in the female pelvis. Am Coll obstet Gynecol Tech Bull 47:1–4

Fisher MS (1976) Metastasis to the esophagus. Gastrointest Radiol 1:249–251

Fox H, Langley FA (1976) Tumors of the ovary. Heinemann, London, ch 12

Gaulayev B, Sherman Y, Diamant Y (1984) A case of triple primary gynecological malignancy. Gynecol Oncol 18:257–260

Gravlee LC (1969) Jet-irrigation method for the diagnosis of endometrial adenocarcinoma. Obstet Gynecol 34:168

Hricak H, Lacey C, Schrick E et al. (1985) Gynecologic masses: value of magnetic resonance imaging. Am J Obstet gynecol 153:31–37

Joelsson I, Levine RU, Moberger G (1971) Hysteroscopy as an adjunct in determining the extent of carcinoma of the endometrium. Am J Obstet Gynecol 111:696–702

Jones HW (1975) Treatment of adenocarcinoma of the endometrium. Obstet Gynecol Surv 30:147–169

Karlen JR, Sternberg LB, Abbott JN (1972) Carcinoma of the endometrium co-existing Pregnancy. Obstet Gynecol 40:334–339

Kawada CY, An-Foraker SH (1979) Screening for endometrial carcinoma. Clin Obstet Gynecol 22:713–728

Kempson RL, Pokorny GE (1968) Adenocarcinoma of the endometrium in women aged forty and younger. Cancer 21:650–662

Knapp RH, Fritz SR, Reiman HM (1982) Primary embryonal carcinoma and choriocarcinoma of the mediastinum. Arch Pathol Lab Med 106:507–509

Koss LG, Schreiber K, Moussouris M et al. (1982) Endometrial carcinoma and its precursors: detection and screening. Clin Obstet Gynecol 25:49–61

Kottmeier HL (1953) Carcinoma of the female genitalia. Williams and Wilkins, Baltimore

Kurman RJ, Craig JM (1972) Endometrioid and clear cell carcinoma of the ovary. Cancer 29: 1653–1664

Lang JH Wu BZ, Tang MY (1978) Endometrial carcinoma, a clinico-pathologic analysis of 108 cases, J Chin Obstet Gynecol 13:6–12

Latrop JC, Wachtel TJ, Meissner CF (1978) Uterine choriocarcinoma fourteen years following bilateral tubal ligation. Obstet Gynecol 51:477–482

Lawrence DW (1984) Gynecologic pathology specialty conference. International Academy of Pathology, San Francisco

Lewis BV, Stallworthy JA, Cordell R (1970) Adenocarcinoma of the body of the uterus. J Obstet Gynecol Br Commonw 77:343–348

Linden M, Roger V (1982) Diagnosis of endometrial carcinoma using the Mi-Mark(R) Helix Sampling Technique. Acta Obstet Gynecol Scand 61:227

Lindermann HJ (1972) The use of CO_2 in the uterine cavity for hysteroscopy. Int J Fertil 7221–224

Lindemann HJ (1974) CO_2 hysteroscopy, diagnosis and treatment. In: Phillips JM, Keith L (eds) Gynecological laparoscopy. Symposia specialists, Miami, p 299

Li SY (1988) Prognosis of endometrial carcinoma. In: Li SY (ed) Endometrial carcinoma. People's Medical Publishing House, Beijing, 169–189

MacMahon B, Austin JH (1969) Association of carcinoma of the breast and corpus uteri. Cancer 23:275–280

Malkasian GD, Annegers JF, Fountain KS (1980) Carcinoma of the endometrium: stage I. Am J Obstet Gynecol 136:872–888

Marinaccio L, Mazzarella L (1967) Gravindansa con parto a termine in soggetto affetto da adenoacanthoma dell 'endometrio'. Cancro (Italy) 20:582–601

Matlock DL, Salem FA, Charles EH, Savage EW (1982) Synchronous multiple neoplasms of the upper female genital tract. Gynecol Oncol 13:271–277

Mattingly RF (1985) Malignant tumors of the uterus. In: Mattingly RF, Thompson JD (eds) Telinde's operative gynecology, 6th edn. Lippincott, Philadelphia, 845–876

McKechnie C, Fechner RE (1971) Choriocarcinoma and adenocarcinoma of the esophagus with gonadotropin secretion. Cancer 27:694–702

Moertel CG, Dockerty MB, Baggenstass AH (1961) Multiple primary malignant neoplasms. II. Tumors of different tissue or organs. Cancer 14:231–237

Mold JW (1969) Benign solid teratoma of uterus. J Pathol 99:173–175

Morris M, Noumoff J, Beckman EM, Bigelow B (1985) Endometrial carcinoma presenting with ascites. Gynecol Oncol 21:186–195

Munnell EW, Taylor HC (1949) Ovarian carcinoma. Am J Obstet Gynecol 58:943–959

Musumeci R, DePalo G, Couti V et al. (1980) Are retroperitoneal lymph node metastases a major problem in endometrial adenocarcinoma? Cancer 46:1887–1892

Nicholson GW (1956) Studies on tumor formation. XXI. A polypoid teratoma of the uterus. Guy's Hosp Rep 105:157–189

Obe JA, Rosen N, Koss LG (1983) Primary choriocarcinoma of the urinary bladder: report of a case with probable epithelial origin. Cancer 52:1405–1409

Pacifico E, Miraglia M, Miraglia F (1982) Diagnosis of endometrial carcinoma and its precusors by means of cytologic examination of jet-washing material. Acta Cytol 26:630–632

Park CH, Reid JD (1980) Adenocarcinoma of the colon with choriocarcinoma in its metastasis. Cancer 46:570–575

Pyrah RD, Redman TF (1968) Teratoma of the uterus with an associated congenital anomaly. J Pathol Bacteriol 95:291–295

Requard CK, Wicks JD, Mettler FA Jr (1981) Ultrasonography in the staging of endometrial adenocarcinoma. Radiology 140:781–785

Richard RM, Barron BAA (1969) Follow-up study of cervical dysplasia. Am J Obstet Gynecol 105:386–393

Rutledge FN (1974) The role of radical hysterectomy in adenocarcinoma of the endometrium. Gynecol Oncol 2:331–347

Saigo PE, Rosen PP (1981) Mammary carcinoma with "choriocarcinomatous" features. Am J Surg Pathol 5:773–778

Saigo PE, Rosen PP, Brigati DJ et al. (1981) Primary gastric choriocarcinoma: an immunohistological study. Am J Surg Pathol 5:333–342

Sandstrom RE, Welch WR, Green TH Jr (1978) Adenocarcinoma of the endometrium in pregnancy. Obstet Gynecol 53:73S–76S

Savage J, Subby W, Okagaki T (1987) Adenocarcinoma of the endometrium with trophoblastic differentiation and metastases as choriocarcinoma: a case report. Gynecol Oncol 26:257–262

Schoenberg BS, Greenberg RA, Eisenberg H (1969) Occurrence of certain multiple primary cancer in females. JNCI 43:15–32

Schoenberg BS (1977) Multiple primary malignant neoplasms: the Connecticut experience 1935–1964. Springer, Vienna New York

Schottenfeld D, Berg J (1971) Incidence of multiple primary cancer. IV. Cancer of the female breast and genital organs. JNCI 46:161–170

Schueller EF, Kirol PM (1966) Prognosis in endometrial carcinoma of the ovary. Obstet Gynecol 27:850–858

Schumann EA (1927) Observation upon the coexistence of carcinoma fundus uteri and pregnancy. Trans Amer Gynecol Soc 52:245–256

Schwartz Z, Ohel G, Birkenfeld A et al. (1985) Second primary malignancy in endometrial carcinoma patients. Gynecol Oncol 22:40–45

Scully RE, Richardson GS, Barlow JF (1966) The development of malignancy in endometriosis. Clin Obstet Gynecol 9:384–411

Sedagal E, Iversen OE (1983) Endoscann, a new endometrial cell sampler. Br J Obstet Gynaecol 90:266–271

Silverberg E (1975) Gynecologic cancer: statistical and epidemiological information. American Cancer Society

Sugimoto O (1975) Hysteroscopic diagnosis of endometrial carcinoma. Am J Obstet Gynecol 121:105–113

Sugimoto O (1981) Diagnostic hysteroscopy in gynecologic oncology. In: Coppleson M, (ed) Fundamental principles and clinical practice. Churchill Livingstone, Edinburgh p 229–239

Surwit EA, Fowler WC Jr, Rogoff EE (1978) Stage II carcinoma of the endometrium: an analysis of treatment. Obstet Gynecol 52:97–99

Suzuki A, Konishi I, Okamura H, Nanashima N (1984) Adenocarcinoma of the endometrium associated with intrauterine pregnancy. Gynecol Oncol 18:261–269

Tak WK, Anderson B, Vardi JR et al. (1977) Myometrial invasion and hysterography in endometrial carcinoma. Obstet Gynecol 50:159–165

Thickman I, Kressel H, Gussman D et al. (1984) Nuclear magnetic resonance imaging in gynecology. Am J Roentgenol 141:835–840

Tyagi SP, Saxena K, Rivi R, Langley FA (1979) Foetal remnants in the uterus and their relation to other uterine heterotopia. Histopathology 3:339

Valle RF, Sciarra JJ (1979) Current status of hysteroscopy in gynecologic practice. Fertil Steril 32:619–632

Vongtama V, Kurohara SS, Badib AO, Webster JH (1970) Second primary cancers of endometrial carcinoma. Cancer 26:842–846

Wall JA, Lucci JA Jr (1953) Adenocarcinoma of the corpus uteri and pelvic tuberculosis complicating pregnancy. Obstet Gynecol 2:629–635

Wallin TE, Malkasian GD, Gaffey TA et al. (1984) Stage II cancer of the endometrium: pathologic and clinical study. Gynecol Oncol 18:1–17

Wallingford AJ (1934) Cancer of the body of the uterus complicating pregnancy. Amer J Obstet Gynecol 27:224–231

Walsh JW, Brewer WH, Schneider V (1980) Ultrasound diagnosis in diseases of the uterine corpus and cervix. Semin Ultrasound 1:30–40

Warren S, Gates O (1932) Multiple primary tumors: a survey of the literature and a statistical study. Am J Cancer 16:1358–1414

Westmann AA (1934) Case of simultaneous pregnancy and cancer of the corpus uteri. Acta Obstet Gynecol Scand 14:191–194

White AJ, Buchsbaum HJ, Rodman NF (1973) Accuracy of the Gravlee Jet washer in detecting endometrial adenocarcinoma. Am J Obstet Gynecol 116:1169–1170

White TGEA (1955) Chorion-epithelioma of the uterus in a postmenopausal woman. J Obstet Gynecol Br Emp 62:372

Wurzel J, Brooks JJ (1981) Primary gastric choriocarcinoma. Cancer 48:2756–2761

Wu BZ, Tang MY, Lang JH (1982) Endometrial carcinoma. In: Lin QZ (ed) Gynecologic oncology. People's Medical Publishing House, Beijing, 85–104

Zarian LP, Berliner L, Redmond P (1983) Metastatic endometrial carcinoma to the esophagus. Am J Gastroenterol 78:9–11

4 Treatment of Endometrial Carcinoma

4.1 Historical Review

Nearly one century has passed since Thomas Cullen, in his book *Cancer of the Uterus* published in 1900, described the treatment of endometrial carcinoma with abdominal hysterectomy and bilateral salpingo-oophorectomy and recommended vaginal hysterectomy only in the very obese or medically indigent patients. In the 1920s, Healy was one of the first to study the effects of radiation alone and in combination with surgery in the treatment of endometrial carcinoma. It confirmed that poorly differentiated carcinoma was more difficult to be treated successfully. In 1936, Arneson compared radiation plus surgery with surgery and radiation alone and found that the combination of radiation, followed 3–6 weeks later by hysterectomy was the best method to treat cancer of the corpus uteri and yielded improved 5-year survival. In 1941 Heyman developed a technique of packing the uterus with multiple capsules of radium prior to hysterectomy and showed approximately 60% 5-year survivals in stage I patients.

In the late 1940's, Brunschwig and Murphy (1954) popularized the use of radical hysterectomy for endometrial carcinoma. They suggested the removal of possible lymph node metastasis, paravaginal tissue, and the upper portion of the vagina. Although results were good, morbidity was high. During this period, other investigators were also interested in radical surgery for the treatment of endometrial carcinoma. In 1956, Javert and Douglas recommended exploratory laparotomy without irradiation in operable patients with endometrial cancer based on their own study and a literature review. Hysterectomy and complete pelvic lymphadenectomy were carried out if no metastases were noted on intraabdominal evaluation. Selective lymphadenectomy was advised if obvious metastases were found. Even though selective lymphadenectomy was worthless from the standpoint of cure when the nodes were positive, lymph node data might be important in predicting the use of postoperative external irradiation and assessing prognosis. Selective or complete lymphadenectomy did not increase morbidity or mortality. The overall survival did not seem to be greater in the surgery combined with preoperative irradiation group than in those individuals who were treated with surgery only. The use of postoperative external irradiation might be effective in patients found to have positive nodes or pelvic extension. In 1974, Rutledge summarized and analyzed the role of radical surgery in the treatment of stage I endometrial carcinoma. From his review, the incidence of pelvic node involvement was shown to be 10%–12% in stage I disease. Patients treated with such radical surgery had the same 5-year survival as those treated with other modalities, and had, however, decreased vaginal recurrence. In Rutledge's opinion, neither the frequency of positive nodes nor the decreased vaginal recurrence justified routine lymphadenectomy in the treatment of stage I disease. At the same time, several studies have shown that radiation with either radium or external therapy, in combination with simple hysterectomy, will yield the same low incidence of vaginal recurrence. After this, most authors agreed that radical hysterectomy and pelvic lymphadenectomy are not indicated in stage I endometrial carcinoma but in stage II endometrial carcinoma.

During the 1940s and the following decades, great emphasis has been placed on the use of preoperative irradiation. The techniques of preoperative irradiation were used including Heyman's packing, standard uterine tube, vaginal ovoids, and external irradiation. In theory, the irradiation should have minimized the viability of cancer cells which might be disseminated at operation and sterilized subclinical vaginal metastases. Many reports were presented indicating that patients treated with preoperative irradiation had less residual disease in the uterus at the time of hysterectomy. In 1975, Jones surveyed the extensive literature from the 1950s to the 1970s and noted that the 5-year survival rate for patients treated with surgery only was the same as that following radiation plus surgery (Table 4.1).

Unfortunately, the vast majority of these reports were not evaluated in regard to grade of tumor or myometrial involvement. Therefore, the overall survival rates were not corrected by the prognostic factors.

More recently, interest has focussed on the incidence of recurrence and 5-year survival after either combined therapy with preoperative or postoperative radiation and surgery or surgery alone. A considerable amount of data has been published concerning the prognostic factors and prognosis in endometrial carcinoma. In general, it appears that surgery combined with preoperative or postoperative irradiation may reduce the incidence of vaginal recurrence and parametrial and pelvic lymph node metastases and increase the 5-year survival. This is particularly true for the patients with poorly differentiated carcinoma or deeper myometrial invasion (Tables 4.2, 4.3).

From recent studies, it has been suggested that surgery is the cornerstone in the treatment of stage I and II endometrial carcinoma, and adjuvant irradiation can only be given, based on hysterectomy specimen examination, if there is poorly differentiated carcinoma or deeper myometrial invasion.

For many years, endometrial carcinoma was considered less malignant than other genital malignancies and could be cured with simple total hysterectomy and bilateral salpingo-oophorectomy. As a result, endometrial carcinoma was called "toma" endometrioma. Although the prognosis of endometrial carcinoma is one of the most favorable of all gynecologic malignancies, the 5-year survival rate given in the latest FIGO Annual Report (1985) for almost 13 581 cases throughout the world is only 67.7% (Table 4.4). These are far from satisfactory results.

Table 4.1. Comparison of 5-year survival results using surgery alone and radiation plus surgery in the treatment of endometrial carcinoma. (Adapted from Jones 1975)

	Surgery alone		Combined therapy	
	No. patients	Five-year survival (%)	No. patients	Five-year survival (%)
Webb	43	65	79	71
Graham	103	70	135	64
Boutselis	19	64	130	66
Javert	101	65	209	68
Davis	167	46	238	56
Gusberg	178	66	217	81
Dobbie	236	81	384	79
Carmichael	140	85	193	81
Copenhaver	141	79	43	77
Wade	43	75	156	86
Burr	36	78	112	82
Geisler	22	82	99	86
Nilsen	97	84	262	85
Sall	198	82	46	72
Vongtama	50	76	327	85
Graham	33	64	90	78
Joslin	280	79	230	84
Beiler	68	79	64	90
Moltz	83	72	68	81
Shah	37	63	80	72
Wentham	98	70	119	68
Monson	179	92	322	92
Silverberg	40	70	76	79
Total patients	2392		3679	
Total survivors	1794		2886	
Average 5-year survival		75		78

During the past 30 years, many reports on endometrial carcinoma have increased our knowledge of the clinicopathologic characteristics of this tumor and have indicated several reasons which are of prognostic significance. We analyzed the following reasons which affect the improvement of 5-year survival rates:

1. Since the majority of patients with endometrial carcinoma have early lesions at the time of diagnosis, a cure rate of approximately 70% can be achieved with surgery and/or radiotherapy. These results make gynecologic oncologists consider this neoplasms a "benign malignancy" and slow down the development of new and more effective modalities of treatment.

Table 4.2. Survival in stage I carcinoma of the endometrium comparing grade and treatment. (Adapted from Creasman and Weed 1981)

	GI		GII		GIII	
	S	S + R	S	S + R	S	S + R
Wharam	80/82	14/14	63/69	60/69	5/9	15/26
Frick	78/88	78/86	7/10	25/36	3/5	9/14
Salazar	10/12	10/11	13/14	38/42	12/17	67/81
Total	168/182	102/111	83/93	123/147	20/31	91/121
	(92.3%)	(91.8%)	(89.2%)	(83.6%)	(64.5%)	(75.2%)

S, surgery; R, radiation therapy.

Table 4.3. Survival in stage I carcinoma of endometrium comparing depth of invasion and treatment. (Adapted from Frick HC et al. 1973)

Depth of invasion	Surgery only	Surgery and radiation
No tumor	11/12 (91.6%)	27/28 (96.4%)
Endometrium and inner muscle	69/80 (86.2%)	49/64 (76.5%)
Mid or outer muscle	8/11 (72.7%)	36/44 (81.8%)

Table 4.4. Carcinoma of the endometrium. Review of the 5-year survival rate by stage reported from 1962 to 1978. (Adapted from FIGO 1985, p. 126)

Stage	Patients treated in 1962–1968	1969–1972	1973–1975	1976–1978
I	71.9	73.6	74.2	75.1
II	49.7	55.7	57.4	57.8
III	30.7	31.3	29.2	30.0
IV	9.3	9.2	9.6	10.6
TOTAL	63.0	65.4	66.6	67.7

2. In recent years a number of studies have indicated several important prognostic factors such as histologic type, histologic differentiation, cervical involvement, depth of myometrial invasion, and regional lymph node metastases. These prognostic factors are linked to the recurrence of endometrial carcinoma. Therefore, it is necessary to have more effective individualized modalities of treatment for these patients. It is usually reported that patients

were originally assigned to stage I or stage II, in whom subclinical extra-uterine or extrapelvic extension was revealed either by the surgeon at the time of operation or by the pathologist when examining the operative specimen. According to the definition these cases do not belong to clinical stage III or IV. If they are included in clinical stage I or II when reported, the survival rate should decline. Because subclinically or microscopically detectable extra-uterine or extrapelvic spread has a severe impact on the prognosis of patients of endometrial carcinoma, a surgicopathologic staging has been considered.

3. Once the disease spread outside the uterus or the pelvis, it is difficult to treat it successfully with surgery and/or radiotherapy, and only systemic therapy with hormonal or nonhormonal cytotoxic chemotherapy is left. However, experience with the systemic therapeutic schedule is limited. The rationale of surgery for the primary tumor in patients with extrapelvic tumor spread is still controversial; some authors agree that surgery of the primary tumor can achieve local control of the disease while others consider that total surgical eradication of the disease, in most cases combined with additional radio-therapy, leaves patients with a very limited chance of cure with a more than a 50% recurrence rate. The amount of initial tumor seems to be of little importance and subclinical spread must, therefore, be regarded as a sign of general dissemination.

4. Recurrent endometrial carcinoma received little attention in the past; as a consequence no more effective management has been found for treating these patients, most of whom died of recurrent disease.

4.2 Surgical Treatment

4.2.1 Value of Surgical Treatment

About 75% of patients with endometrial carcinoma present with stage I disease, which portends a favorable prognosis and survival. Five-year survival rates in the literature range from 63% to 94% for stage I carcinoma (Beiler et al. 1972; Piver et al. 1979). Surgery is the cornerstone of treatment for stages I and II endometrial carcinoma. Individual postoperative assessment is necessary to decide whether surgery alone is sufficient or whether adjuvant radiation therapy is necessary (Morrow and Schlaerth 1982). Until now the role of surgery in patients with stage III or IV endometrial carcinoma has been controversial. However, surgery should not be overlooked in the management of stage III and IV disease. Although radiotherapy, hormone therapy, and chemotherapy have a major place in the treatment of these patients, surgery as a cytoreductive procedure could be very advantageous. Even the survival for patients with recurrent disease is very poor and varies from 2% to 12% (Aalders et al. 1984). Surgery should also be reserved for local recurrences amenable to surgical removal, especially suburethral or vaginal vault lesions. Isolated, central post-irradiation recurrence of endometrial carcinoma is curable with radical surgery.

4.2.1.1 Stage I

In stage I disease, the operation of choice is a total abdominal hysterectomy, bilateral salpingo-oopherectomy, and selective lymphadenectomy; and post-operative pathologic evaluation of the uterus, cervix adnexae, and lymph nodes is of the utmost importance in deciding whether any adjunctive therapy is needed. Histologic type and grading, degree of myometrial invasion, distance of the lesion from the cervix, microscopic or overt cervical involvement or possible spread to the adnexae, peritoneum, or lymph nodes will be the deciding factors. Adjunctive therapy may involve radiation, hormone therapy, chemotherapy, or a combination of these modalities.

About 75%–96% of patients with stage I endometrial carcinoma could be treated with surgery alone and the 5-year survival rate was about 80% (Declos and Fischer 1969; Frick et al. 1973; Morrow et al. 1973; Berman et al. 1980; Connelly et al. 1982; Kauppila et al. 1982). In the 228 patients with stage I endometrial carcinoma reported by Li (1988) from the Cancer Institute Hospital, Beijing, 87.3% were treated with surgery alone. Since the majority of all endometrial carcinoma is stage I, the prognostic factors mentioned above would seem even more pertinent in individualizing management.

4.2.1.2 Stage II

The recommended methods of treatment for patients with stage II endometrial carcinoma vary from institution to institution, but 65%–80% of patients may be treated primarily with surgery (Declos and Fischer 1969). The primary treatment for occult stage II endometrial carcinoma (a normal cervix with a positive endocervical scrape) is extended hysterectomy with bilateral salpingo-oophorectomy and selective lymphadenectomy. If postoperative pathologic evaluation confirms a positive prognostic factor, adjunctive radiation is necessary. Stage II disease with macroscopic cervical involvement should be managed with intra-cavitary radiotherapy followed by extended hysterectomy or radical hysterectomy or pelvic lymphadenectomy after an interval of 7–10 days with or without adjunctive postoperative radiotherapy.

Li (1988) reported that the 5-year survival in 66 patients with stage II endometrial carcinoma who were treated with surgery in combination with adjunctive radiotherapy was 70%, and the 5-year survival in 39 patients with stage II endometrial carcinoma treated with radiation alone was 41%. The difference was statistically significant ($P < 0.05$). This shows that surgery in combination with radiation appears to offer advantages over radiation alone.

4.2.1.3 Advanced Carcinoma (Stage III or Stage IV)

Even the role of surgery in patients with advanced endometrial carcinoma is controversial, as surgical eradication of macroscopic tumor was of major prognostic importance in those patients. The rationale of surgery for the primary tumor in patients with extrauterine or extrapelvic tumor spread is to achieve local control of the disease. Resection of the masses, omentum, enlarged lymph nodes, invaded intestine, as well as removal of the uterus, tubes, and ovaries would seem desirable. After surgical eradication of macroscopic tumor, the patient's response to subsequent therapy with other modalities will be improved and the patient's symptoms such as vaginal bleeding and vaginal discharge will be relieved.

4.2.1.4 Recurrent Carcinoma

When the disease is recurrent, the role of surgery depends on the site, extent of recurrence, and the nature and extent of initial treatment. For example, patients who have been treated with radiation therapy alone and who have recurrent disease in the cervix, uterus, or upper vagina may profit from local extirpation. In the 379 patients with recurrent endometrial carcinoma reported by Aalders et al., only 262 could be treated with various forms of treatment. The survival time of 262 patients treated for recurrent endometrial carcinoma compared with that of 117 patients not treated is significantly different. In 36 months all the untreated patients were dead. At that time, 31% of the treated patients were still alive and at 5 years their survival rate was 13% (Aalders et al. 1984). In a group of 75 patients with recurrent endometrial carcinoma, only 45 (60%) were treated. In 6 months, 50% of the untreated patients (15 cases) were dead. At that time, 84.4% of the treated patients were alive and at 5 years the survival rate of treated patients was 24.4% and for the untreated patients 3.4%. Treatment for recurrent endometrial carcinoma may be abandoned only when the disease is too extensive and the medical condition of the patients is deteriorating too rapidly. Otherwise the active treatment should be given (Li 1988).

From those mentioned above, it would seem that the best approach for endometrial carcinoma is to perform surgery initially, because radiation therapy alone is not applicable to all patients. The eradication of cancerous lesions is very important and the true extent of the disease can only be determined post-operatively and individualized treatment will be decided on the basis of pathologic evaluation after surgery.

4.2.2 Common Surgical Approaches for Endometrial Carcinoma

The common surgical approaches are standard total abdominal hysterectomy, extended hysterectomy, and radical hysterectomy. Over the past 30 years, however, certain authorities have modified the operations.

4.2.2.1 Standard Total Hysterectomy

This is a total abdominal hysterectomy and bilateral salpingo-oophorectomy, and the extent of the operation is shown in Fig. 4.1. It has been used as a treatment for stage I endometrial carcinoma. Because the majority of patients have stage I endometrial carcinoma, this type of hysterectomy has been the most common surgical approach.

In an effort to prevent vaginal vault recurrences, a variety of techniques to close the cervical os prior to the hysterectomy have been used. In order to avoid possible spillage of malignant cells from the fallopian tubes, clamping the uterine cornua or ligating the fallopian fimbriae may also be undertaken (Figs. 4.2, 4.3). During the operation, the surgeon's actions should be as gentle as possible to avoid possible pressure to the uterus. The hysterectomy should always include the removal of adnexa because of the risk of ovarian metastasis. Selected biopsy of the pelvic and paraaortic lymph nodes and selected lymphadenectomy must be included.

4.2.2.1.1 Major Operative Procedure

1. With the abdomen opened and before inserting a retractor or abdominal pack, a sample of 60–100 ml peritoneal fluid should be routinely examined for endometrial carcinoma cells. If no peritoneal fluid is obtainable, 200 ml normal saline solution is injected into the pelvis. After admixture of the fluid in the pelvis, it is withdrawn into a sterile vial containing sodium citrate solution and immediately despatched for cytologic screening.
2. Thorough manual exploration of the pelvic abdominal cavity is an extremely important step which should never be omitted. The main purpose is to detect any extrauterine spread of the tumor. The order of exploration should be as

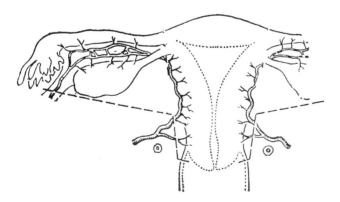

Fig. 4.1. Extent of the incision of total hysterectomy

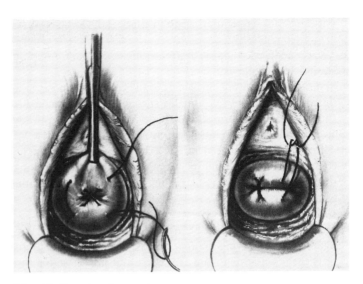

Fig. 4.2. Suturing the cervix

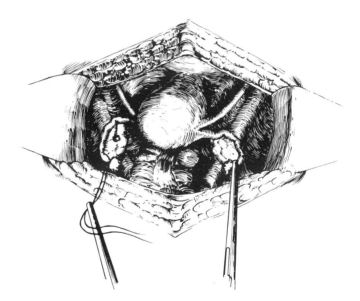

Fig. 4.3. Ligating the distant end of the fallopian tubes to avoid possible spillage of malignant cells

follows: (a) from the upper abdominal organs to the pelvic cavity and (b) from the locations without tumor to the locations with tumor, i.e., from liver, spleen, stomach, kidney, omentum, intestine, mesentery, paraaortic lymph node fields to pelvic lymph nodes, bladder, rectum, adnexa, and uterus. The parametrium, vesicouterine excavation and Douglas pouch should also be examined carefully.

3. The procedure for simple hysterectomy and bilateral salpingo-oophorectomy should be as follows:

a) Clamping, cutting, and ligating the round ligaments (Fig. 4.4). The round ligament tie may be left long for suspension and attached to a clip, elevating the peritoneum laterally to provide improved access to the parametrium.

b) Clamping, cutting, and ligating the infundibulopelvic ligaments (Fig. 4.5). Three clamps are placed on the external side of the ovary and tube, but the residue of the infundibulopelvic ligament should be left long enough in order to prevent the blood vessels from loosening and separating to form hematoma.

c) Incising the uterovesical fold (Figs. 4.6–4.8). The peritoneum of the uterovesical fold is incised at the isthmus level from the cut end of the round ligament in a curving manner across the front of the uterus. The bladder is now easily separated from the cervix and upper vagina by pushing it gently downwards with a swab over the index finger of the right hand until 1 cm down from the external os of the cervix. The pushing of the bladder should be directed to the cervix rather than the bladder in order to avoid rupture of the bladder. If there is bleeding in the uterovesical excavation, which may be produced from the small vessels on the bladder surface, oppression hemostasis should be used.

d) Clamping, cutting, and ligating the uterine arteries (Fig. 4.9). The parametrial tissue is freed until the main vessel of uterine arteries is reached. Three curved Kocher's pressure forceps are placed parallel to the cervix, squeezing the paracervical tissue off the cervix. These clamps should be placed carefully in order to prevent the ureters from becoming injured.

e) Clamping, cutting, and ligating the cardinal and uterosacral ligaments (Figs. 4.10, 4.11). The cardinal ligaments should be clamped along the cervical side and the uterosacral ligaments are usually clamped, cut, and ligated

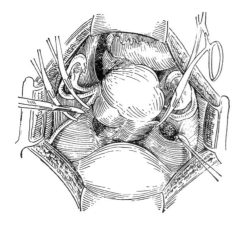

Fig. 4.4. Clamping, cutting, and ligating the round ligament

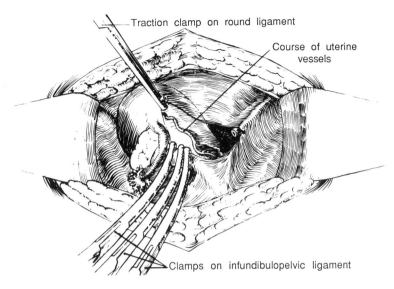

Fig. 4.5. Cutting the infundibulopelvic ligament

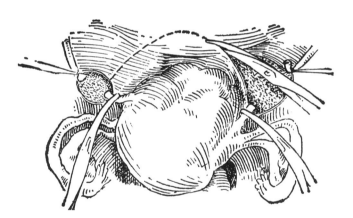

Fig. 4.6. Incising the uterovesical fold

together with the cardinal ligaments. If the uterus is clearly bound, con-
tracture of uterosacral ligaments, clamping, cutting, and ligation of these
ligaments should be undertaken separately.

f) Clamping the vaginal angles, opening the vagina, and removing the uterus.
Clamps should be placed so that they reach the vaginal angle but do not
include any vaginal epithelium (Fig. 4.12). The uterus is drawn up; a knife is
plunged into the anterior fornix; and the knife blade is then run to the right
and to the left around the vagina until the posterior fornix is incised and the

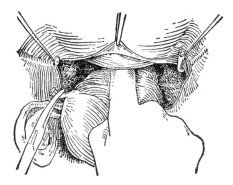

Fig. 4.7. Separating the bladder

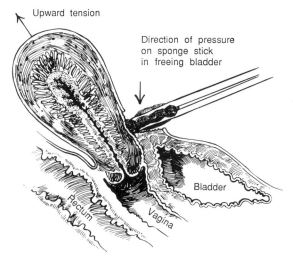

Fig. 4.8. Blunt separation of the bladder from the lower segment of the uterus and cervix

uterus removed. The cervix must be incised totally. The entire circumference of the vagina should be visible and the upper edge of the vagina must be sterilized with iodine solution then closed using continuous gut suture. If suspension is necessary, the pedicle of the vaginal angle should be stitched on the round ligament cut (Fig. 4.13).

g) Closing the abdominal peritonium. Any bleeding which is present should be checked. The peritoneum is reconstituted using a continuous suture, beginning at one side, and attaching the central part of the peritoneum to the apex of the vault to obliterate space.

h) Closing the abdominal cavity.

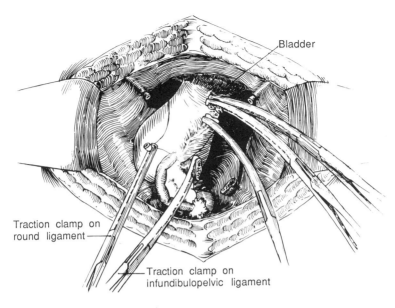

Fig. 4.9. Clamping and cutting the uterine artery

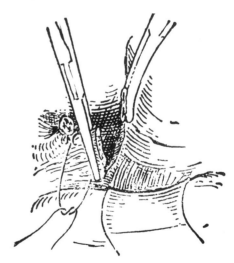

Fig. 4.10. Penetrating suture
of the cardinal ligament

4.2.2.1.2 Preoperative Preparation and Postoperative Treatment

Preoperative Preparation

1. Obesity, hypertension, and diabetes are frequently associated with endometrial cancers. Patients who are obese or associated with hypertension and
   diabetes are immediately at high risk of anesthetic and surgical complications.

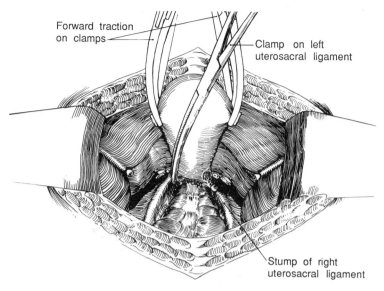

Fig. 4.11. Clamping the uterosacral ligament

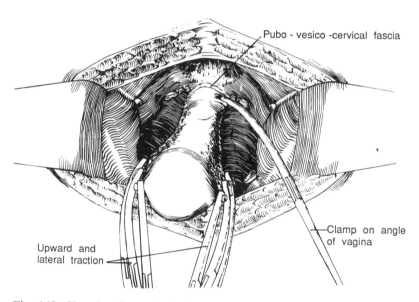

Fig. 4.12. Clamping the vaginal edge

For all these conditions, the physician should take expert advice, asking colleagues in the relevant specialties to examine patients with significant problems. The physician should discuss the patient with the anesthetist.

2. The patient and her relatives must give consent for the operation to be performed in the light of full knowledge of the course of therapy.

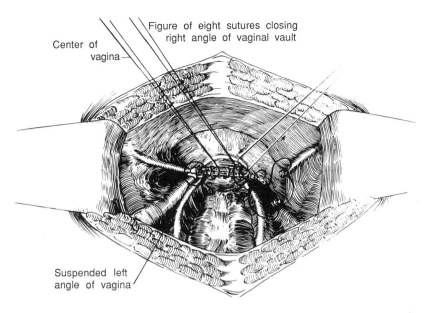

Fig. 4.13. Suspending the vaginal vault

3. At least three consecutive days of vaginal irrigation should be given before the operation.
4. A quantity of 400–800 ml fresh blood should be prepared for transfusion.
5. The most important part of skin preparation is for the operation field to be shaved 1 day prior to operation. More extensive bowel preparation slould consist of enema three times on the evening prior to operation. This enema may be repeated in the morning of operation if there has not been a good result.
6. In the morning of the operation, the vagina should be irrigated and the cervical surface and vaginal wall swabbed with 75% alcohol. A Foley catheter is left in situ. The preoperative drugs for anesthesia should be given according to prescription. Generally, 0.2 g sodium luminal is given intramuscularly 1/2 h before the operation.

Postoperative Treatment

1. A fast is undertaken for 2–3 days until aerofluxus appears and then the patient changes onto a liquid, soft, and routine diet
2. Sedatives should be ordered to keep the patient relatively comfortable for the 1st day of operation. In general, dolantin may be used in the dosage of 50–100 mg i.m. and given every 6 h or p.r.n.

3. The use of prophylactic antibiotics in the postoperative period is controversial. However, the authors of this monograph prefer routine antibiotics in the form of penicillin and streptomycin (800 000 u penicillin and 0.5 g streptomycin twice daily) intramuscularly for 6 days postoperatively.
4. A Foley catheter inserted before surgery is left in the bladder for 2 days following the operation. If there is hematuria, the catheter could be left there longer.
5. The general condition of the patient should be carefully monitored in order to prevent immediate postoperative complications. Because the majority of patients with endometrial carcinoma are old women, attention should be paid to prevent complications of the pulmonary, circulatory, and urinary system. Patients with endometrial carcinoma usually have complications with diabetes mellitus, and an optimal dose of insulin should be given according to the routine treatment of diabetes mellitus in order to correct the concentration of blood sugar and prevent acidosis.
6. External bleeding through the vagina becomes apparent immediately after the operation is concluded. If the bleeding is slight, it can usually be controlled by putting a purse string at the apex of the vagina. If profuse vaginal bleeding occurs, this indicates the operator has failed to include one or more of the vessels in suturing the vagina. It should be transfixed with a figure-of-eight suture. Bleeding may also occur 10–14 days after the operation. Slight bloody discharge in this period of convalescence is common. Such hemorrhage results from absorption of chromic catgut causing the oozing of blood. Any remedial action is unnecessary.
7. If postoperative adjuvant radiation is necessary, it should be started 10–14 days after the operation.

4.2.2.2 Extended Hysterectomy

Extended hysterectomy is applicable to occult stage II endometrial carcinoma (a normal cervix with a positive endocervical scrape). An effective extended hysterectomy is only possible if the ureters are dissected from the ureteral tunnels and displaced laterally to allow the removal of an adequate area of the parametrium and vaginal vault. This is the most important step in extended hysterectomy and is the sole difference between it and simple hysterectomy. The ureters are dissected and exposed down to 5–6 cm from the level of the ovarian pedicle. The bladder is pushed well down off the front of the cervix and upper vagina and the peritoneum is swept laterally to expose the roof of the ureteral tunnel on each side. The aim of the operation is to take as much of the parametrium and the vault of the vagina as possible. The incidence of complications following this procedure is very low and the ureteral fistula occurred only very rarely.

In 1972, Milton and Metters presented their data and compared the 5-year survival rate of endometrial carcinomas treated with simple hysterectomy and extended hysterectomy. The 5-year survival rate was 75.7% for patients treated with simple hysterectomy and 91.4% for those treated with extended hysterectomy. The recurrence rate may also be reduced by extended hysterectomy.

4.2.2.3 Radical Hysterectomy

The area resected should include the uterus, adnexa, parametrium, upper part of the vagina, and pelvic groups of lymph nodes which contain the external iliac, internal iliac, obturator and deep inguinal group and should be used for overt stage II or poorly differentiated (G_3) endometrial carcinoma (Fig. 4.14).

In this operation, the essential steps are as follows:

1. Exposure of the ureters. The uterus is lifted upwards and forwards with forceps on the broad ligaments and each ureter is recognized extraperitoneally as it lies medial to the corresponding ovarian pedicle. It is steadied with dissecting forceps while the peritoneum is incised just lateral to it. Then the ureter is dissected out and marked with a tape for identification. The ureters should be handled gently, otherwise too may vessels are damaged and the blood supply to the ureters is affected (Fig. 4.15).
2. Dissection of the common iliac, external iliac, hypogastric, obturator, and deep inguinal lymph nodes. Lymph node dissection should consist of the removal of all visible lymph nodes, lymph vessels, and areolar and adipose tissue from the bifurcation of the aorta down to the point at which the uterine artery was tied. The external iliac artery and vein are exposed and the ureter is slightly pushed to the medial line. The fascia over the iliopsoas muscle is now picked up and incised along the line of external artery, taking care not to damage the genitofemoral nerve (Fig. 4.16).

The common iliac lymph nodes with adipose tissue and the perivascular sheet should be removed first. The line of dissection continues along the

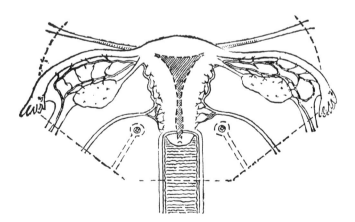

Fig. 4.14. Extent of incision of radical hysterectomy

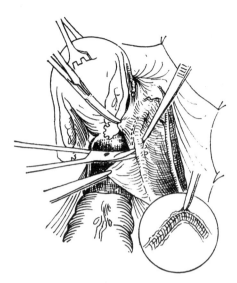

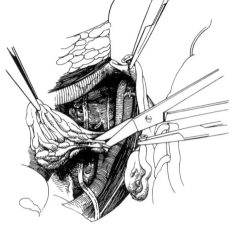

Fig. 4.15. Exposing the ureter

Fig. 4.16. Completing the pelvic lymph node dissection in the obturator fossa

length of the external iliac artery, producing a sheet of fascia and nodal tissue which will leave the arteries clean from the bifurcation of the artery to the inguinal ligament. If it is possible to roll the vessels round, all the nodal tissues may be removed en bloc. This dissection dips below the external iliac vein so that the obturator fossa can be emptied of all nodal materials, taking care not to damage the obturator vessels and nerves (Fig. 4.17). At the upper end of the dissection, the sheet of tissue separated is continued down the hypogastric artery, taking great care not to damage the ureter (Fig. 4.18).

3. Ligating and cutting the uterine artery at the level of branching from the hypogastric artery. The obliterated umbilical artery is lifted up and the uterine artery isolated. Double ligature is applied and the artery is severed (Figs. 4.19, 4.20).

4. Opening the pararectal and paravesical fossa: The peritoneum is cut between the sacrum and rectum parallel to and medially of the upper edge of the uterosacral ligament. The best way to separate the rectum from the rectal pillars is to grasp it with fine-toothed tissue forceps, lifting and pulling it medially. Now the lateral posterior part of the rectrorectal space as well as the pararectal space adjacent to the uterosacral ligament can easily be entered with a finger.

Advancing into the retrorectal space parallel to the rectal wall, one exposes the stalked uterosacral ligament at its origin on the sacrum. The entire rectrorectal space is usually exposed spontaneously when the uterosacral ligament is clamped and cut close to the pelvic wall (Figs. 4.21, 4.22). It contains delicate connective and lymphatic tissue which can be removed without difficulty.

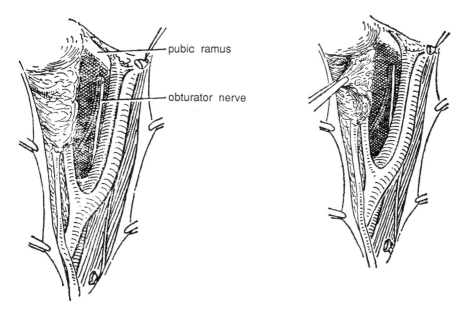

Fig. 4.17 (*left*). Obturator nerve and vessels

Fig. 4.18 (*right*). Dissecting the lymph nodes from the internal iliac vessels

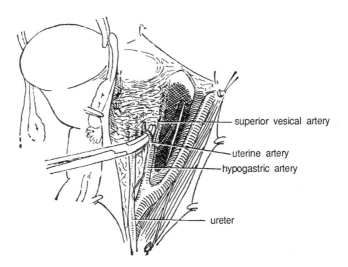

Fig. 4.19. Separating the uterine artery

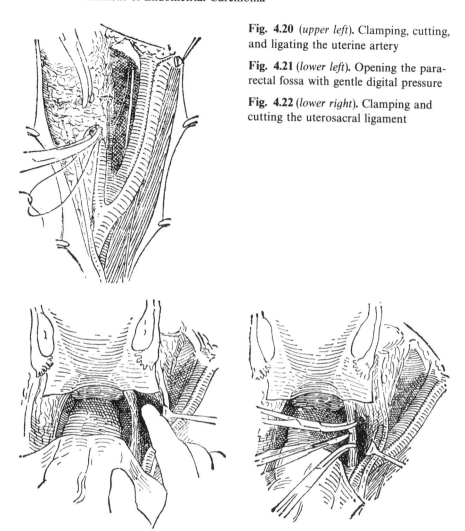

Fig. 4.20 (*upper left*). Clamping, cutting, and ligating the uterine artery

Fig. 4.21 (*lower left*). Opening the pararectal fossa with gentle digital pressure

Fig. 4.22 (*lower right*). Clamping and cutting the uterosacral ligament

   The space of fine connective tissue in front of the cardinal ligament (paravesical space) is now dissected bluntly. The lateral umbilical ligament is pulled laterally. The cardinal ligament which separates the paravesical and pararectal fossa is carefully lifted with a curved clamp so that its upper part can be clamped and cut. It is now possible to separate the rectum from the vagina as far as possible. The delicate connective and lymphatic tissue can be removed (Figs. 4.23, 4.24).

5. Opening the ureteral canal and freeing the lower part of the ureters: In front of the bladder near the entrance of the ureter, some connective tissue should be left on the ureter and bladder so that the ureter is surrounded by a kind of lateral half-cone of tissue. The cone at the entrance of the ureter into the bladder is actually a half-cone consisting of the lateral part of the vesico-

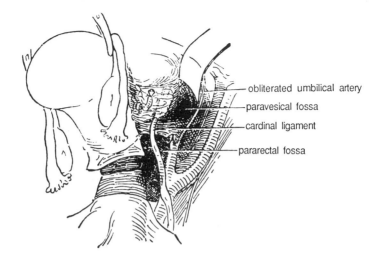

Fig. 4.23. Opening the paravesical fossa

- obliterated umbilical artery
- paravesical fossa
- cardinal ligament
- pararectal fossa

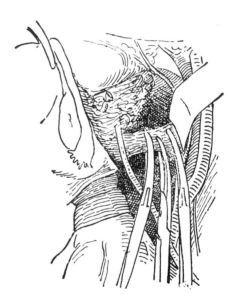

Fig. 4.24. Clamping and incision of the lateral portion of the cardinal ligament adjacent to the lateral pelvic wall

uterine ligament and the adventitia of the ureter. It is preferable to open the medial part of the ureteral canal so that the vesicouterine ligament can be tied and cut near the ureter (Fig. 4.25). Having cut the anterior vesico uterine ligament, the ureters are pushed downward and laterally, so that the posterior vesico-uterine ligament is exposed, clamped, cut, and ligated near the bladder.

Now the bladder and ureter have to be dissected from the paracolpium, which has already been divided. Any paracolpium remaining on the pelvic floor has to

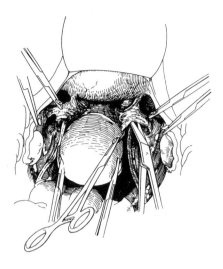

Fig. 4.25. Identifying the ureteral canal

be clamped and cut. The inferior vesical artery and vein and venous vaginal plexus, while dissecting the bladder and the ureter from the paracolpium, should be managed carefully. Using this procedure, the vaginal and paravaginal tissues, 3–4 cm from the external os of the cervix, may be resected.

Controversial ideas exist about the value of radical hysterectomy for the management of patients with endometrial carcinoma. The rationale for radical hysterectomy comes from the incidence of pelvic lymph node metastasis of about 10% in stage I and 36% in stage II (Jones 1975). Radical hysterectomy should also reduce the incidence of vaginal apex recurrence and would seem especially suitable for patients with stage II lesions with macroscopic cervical involvement and a high incidence of nodal metastasis.

However, in the multiple series reporting the use of radical hysterectomy for stage II disease, the 5-year survival rates were 9%–70% (Delclos and Fletcher 1969). A disease-free survival of 83% at 10 years was found in combination radiation and total abdominal hysterectomy for stage II endometrial carcinoma (Kinsella et al. 1980). Therefore better survival statistics with much less morbidity can be obtained with the use of combination radiation and total abdominal hysterectomy than with the use of radical hysterectomy for stage II endometrial carcinoma.

In the series reported by Lewis (1970) and of the seven patients with positive pelvic lymph nodes who died of cancer, only one had developed a pelvic recurrence. This suggested that patients with pelvic lymph nodal metastasis from endometrial carcinoma already have a high incidence of extrapelvic disease at the time of their original therapy. The survival rates obtained by radical hysterectomy are equal, but not superior, to those obtained by less radical surgery.

The morbidity associated with radical hysterectomy is significant. Park et al. (1974) reported a 24% incidence of major operative complications in patients undergoing "extended hysterectomy." The technical difficulties of radical hysterectomy are often increased by the frequent obesity of the patient with endometrial carcinoma and the likelihood of associated diabetes, hypertension, and advanced age which cause the poor medical condition of these patients. Vaginal hysterectomy for endometrial carcinoma has several advantages. Since this procedure is often shorter and less traumatic than abdominal hysterectomy, it has generally been selected for patient who are obese or poor in medical condition. This procedure has better operability than the abdominal procedure. However, due to the inability to explore the abdomen and the difficulty in removing the adnexae, vaginal hysterectomy for endometrial carcinoma is not generally recommended. It is limited to those unsuitable for the abdominal approach.

4.2.3 Problems of Surgery

4.2.3.1 Preliminary Suture of the Cervix

Preliminary suture of the cervix may be an advantage. Certainly, cancer cells are broken loose by manipulation and may become implanted. This was suggested by McGrew et al. (1954), who, in the treatment of cancer of the colon, found that well-preserved and possibly viable cancer cells were present in smears made of the contents of the removed specimens. In 42% of the proximal ends and in 65% of the distal ends, cells were found. The same kind of spill must occur during hysterectomy.

Probable mechanisms of vaginal recurrence of endometrial carcinoma following completion of primary therapy have been described, which include: (a) direct implantation of tumor cells at surgery and (b) retrograde lymphatic or venous spread.

The mechanism of direct implantation, while plausible from a theoretical standpoint, has not been proven, as no study has been reported which shows a decrease in vaginal recurrence or improvement in 5-year survival with preoperative suture of the cervix (Jones 1975; Morrow and Townsend 1981). Truskett and constable (1968) studied the correlation between the vault recurrence rate and preoperative irradiation. It is assumed that those who have preoperative irradiation and a sterile uterus at operation are not suitable for local implants, and it would seem from these results that cancer cells present in the paravaginal tissues or lymphatics at the time of operation are more important than implantation.

Some authors have considered the preoperative closure of the cervix to be unnecessary (Creasman and Weed 1981; DuToit 1985). In the Cancer Institute Hospital, Beijing, preoperative suture of the cervix has also been the routine procedure, especially in patients with an enlarged and soft uterus. If the uterine cavity was occupied by neoplasm, preoperative suture of the cervix can prevent spillage of tumor cells from the cervix.

4.2.3.2 Value of Peritoneal Cytology at Laparotomy

It is generally accepted that a sample of peritoneal fluid should be examined routinely at laparotomy for endometrial carcinoma cells and the result be incorporated in the staging of the disease. However, the value of peritoneal cytology at laparotomy for stage I endometrial carcinoma as a progonostic factor is controversial. The peritoneal fluid is positive for malignancy in 11% –15.5% of patients with endometrial carcinoma (Table 4.5) (Creasman and Rutledge 1971; Creasman et al. 1981; Yazigi et al. 1983).

Creasman et al. (1981) reported positive cytology in 26 of the 167 patients (15.5%) with stage I endometrial carcinoma, and 10 of these patients (34%) developed recurrences as opposed to only 14 out of the 141 patients (10%) with negative cytologic washings.

A retrospective study was performed by Kennedy et al. in 1986 to assess the significance and value of pelvic washings in stage I and II endometrial adenocarcinoma. Of the 163 patients, 6 (3.7%) were positive and 3 (1.8%) had suspected malignant cells. Positive results for each FIGO stage, grade of neoplasm, and depth of myometrial invasion are as follows:

Stage			Grade			Myometrial invasion		
	IA	3/107		I	0/57		None	0/70
	IB	2/37		II	2/73		1/3	3/62
	II	1/19		III	4/33		2/3	1/18
	II	1/19		III	4/33		3/3	2/13

It is concluded that pelvic washings in stage I and II endometrial adenocarcinoma have an extremely limited role in clinical management. The Gynecologic Oncology Group (GOG) presented a preliminary report dealing with the 528 patients for whom all surgical staging data and at least 2 years of follow-up were available. It repeated the pelvic cytology study first reported from the Norwegian Radium Hospital by Dahle in 1956. The frequency of positive pelvic cytology suggested that this could be an important cause of treatment failure and partly answers the perennial question about the source of vaginal cuff recurrence in endometrial carcinoma (Morrow et al. 1986).

Table 4.5. Positive peritoneal cytology in endometrial carcinoma

Series	Year	Patients	Positive cytology (n)	(%)
Creasman and Rutledge	1971	183	21	11.5
Keettel et al.	1974	38	5	13.2
Creasman et al.	1981	167	26	15.5
Yazigi et al.	1983	93	10	11.0

4.2.3.2 Pelvic and Paraaortic Lymph Node Sampling and Resection

It is well known that pelvic and paraaortic lymph nodal metastases are of prime importance in the patient's prognosis. Endometrial carcinoma metastasizes to lymph nodes in a significant number of patients even in stage I disease (Piver et al. 1982). The incidence of pelvic and paraaortic lymph node metastases in stage I endometrial carcinoma is shown in Table 4.6.

Morrow et al. (1973) reviewed the literature over 15 years and noted that in the collected series 10.6% (39/369 cases) of patients with stage I endometrial carcinoma and 36.5% (31/85 cases) with stage II endometrial carcinoma had pelvic node metastases. They found that the incidence of lymph node metastases in patients with cervical involvement was considerably higher. The incidence of lymph node metastases increased when the tumor was more undifferentiated and penetrated further into the myometrium. Table 4.7 shows the correlation between pelvic, paraaortic lymph node metastases and stage, histologic grade, and myometrial invasion.

Table 4.6. Stage I endometrial carcinoma. Status of pelvic and paraaortic lymph nodes

Series	Year	Patients (*n*)	Positive nodes Pelvic nodes (%)	Paraaortic nodes (%)
Lewis et al.	1970	102	11.2	–
Creasman et al.	1976	140	11.4	5.7
Piver et al.	1982	41	–	14.6
Boronow et al.	1984	222	10.4	7.6

Table 4.7. Stage I endometrial carcinoma: clinical stage and histologic grade versus lymph node status. (Adapted from Morrow et al. 1973)

	Positive nodes	
	Pelvic nodes (%)	Paraaorric nodes (%)
Ia	6	4
Ib	18	12
GI	3	2
GII	10	4
GIII	36	28
Endometrial only	4	2
Inner third	12	10
Mid third	10	0
Outer third	43	21

Uterine carcinoma may spread directly to the paraaortic lymph nodes via the lymphatics of the ovarian vessels without involving the pelvic lymph nodes. Henrikson (1949) found that 20.3% of his cases had positive aortic lymph nodes with negative pelvic nodes and Beck and Latour (1963) reported this in 13.6% of their cases.

At present, it is generally accepted that those patients with positive paraaortic lymph nodes would have poor prognosis and eventually die of the disease. It seems that the paraaortic lymph node metastases are more important than the clinical stage in predicting the prognosis of endometrial carcinoma. It is unreliable to ascertain pelvic or paraaortic lymph node metastases with manual exploratory examination only, as the microscopic metastases can only be diagnosed by pathologic examination. Lymph node biopsy and lymphadenectomy should be considered as a rational method for the diagnosis of lymph node metastases. The indications for pelvic or paraaortic lympth node biopsy in endometrial carcinoma are as follows:

1. Those patients with a poorly differentiated lesion, grade III (G III).
2. For those patients with a well or moderately differentiated lesion grade I or grade II, the depth of myometrial invasion and isthmic or cervical involvement should be examined at the time of laparotomy. If there is evidence of deep myometrial invasion or isthmic or cervical involvement, staging internal, external iliac, and paraaortic lymph node biopsy should be undertaken.
3. No matter what the histologic grade is, if a large or suspicious lymph node is encountered at the time of laparotomy, lymph node biopsy should be carried out.

The rationale for pelvic lymphadenectomy in endometrial carcinoma is as follows: Based on frozen section technique, if there is histologic evidence of iliac lymph nodal metastases and the paraaortic lymph nodes are negative for metastases, pelvic lymphadenectomy should be considered. If there is histologic evidence of paraaortic lymph nodal metastases, which probably represents a systemic disease, it is not necessary to perform lymphadenectomy. Adjuvant external radiation to the pelvic and paraaortic lymph nodes may be given. Marking the location of those lymph nodes with radiopaque clips will facilitate postoperative radiotherapy.

4.3 Radiotherapy

4.3.1 Indication and Value

Since its beginning in 1920, radiotherapy and surgery have developed successfully. Radiotherapy has played a major role in the treatment of endometrial carcinoma. Radiotherapy may be used alone, sometimes combined with chemotherapy or hormone therapy, or as an adjuvant to surgery.

4.3.1.1 Radiotherapy Alone

Radiotherapy can be the unique primary treatment modality or combined with other treatment methods such as chemotherapy and hormone therapy. It may be divided into radical or palliative radiation depending upon the expected treatment results. Radiotherapy may be used for patients (a) in stage I and II disease, if surgery is contraindicated or refused by patients; (b) in stage III or IV disease, if the tumor has been extensively invasive and the probability of eradicating disease with surgery is too low, or if the general condition is not good enough to be operated on; and (c) with recurrent disease, if the patient has never received radiation and the tumor has a recurrent location and is not amenable to surgical removal.

4.3.1.2 Radiotherapy as an Adjuvant to Surgery

Preoperative radiation, postoperative radiation, or a combination of pre- and postoperative radiation may be used as an adjuvant to surgery. The aim of this kind of therapy is to reduce the chance of local, lymphatic, and vascular dissemination of cancer at hysterectomy; cure the lymph nodes, structure, and tissue involved within the pelvis and reduce pelvic and vaginal recurrence.

In view of the above, it is clear that radiotherapy does play an important role in the management of endometrial carcinoma. Not only could it be used for all of the stage lesions but it could be used either as a unique treatment modality or as an adjuvant to surgery, either as a radical or a palliative policy. Therefore, radiotherapy is still an important measure in the treatment of endometrial carcinoma.

4.3.2 Intracavitary Irradiation

Intracavitary treatment was fully developed during the period of 1930–1950 in the following two aspects: (a) an evenly distributed dose of radiation throughout the uterine volume and (b) an adequate dose of radiation to the periphery of a deeply invasive tumor.

4.3.2.1 Application of Sources

The correct application of sources is extremely important in order to provide an adequate distribution of radiation to what is often an irregularly shaped intrauterine carcinoma and enlarged uterine cavity. There are four basic types of intrauterine insertion:

4.3.2.1.1 Tandem

This takes the form of a single series of sources forming the basis of the Manchester system. A 25 mg ^{226}Ra source or 75 mCi ^{137}Cs is placed at the fundal end and two or more 10 mg ^{226}Ra sources or 30 mCi ^{137}Cs in the tandem below it. Vaginal ovoids loaded with 10 mg ^{226}Ra or 30 mCi ^{137}Cs are used during one or two insertions lasting 72 h spaced 7 days apart. This delivers a dose of 80 Gy 2 cm from the central tube. In the Cancer Institute Hospital, Beijing, the long, mediate, short intracavitary applicators are loaded with 60, 40, 20 mg ^{137}Cs respectively. The diameter of the applicator is 4.5 mm, which may easily be inserted into the uterine cavity without dilating the cervical canal. The vaginal applicators are of different types and sizes, which are loaded with two to six radiation units, each unit containing 10 mg ^{137}Cs. The type and size of the applicator chosen depends on the size of tumor, the extension of disease, and the width of tumor (Fig. 4.26).

4.3.2.1.2 Hysterostats

In 1965, Strickland developed this technique, which uses a helical spring of flexible steel to form a loop to fit the uterine cavity so that the radioactive sources may suit the uterine cavity. It has not been widely used until now.

4.3.2.1.3 Packing Technique

This method came from Sweden and was greatly advocated by Heyman in 1947. It depends upon packing the uterine cavity tightly with ^{226}Ra or ^{137}Cs capsules (Heyman capsules) in an attempt to raise the 5-year survival rate from 45% to 65% (Heyman 1947).

Heyman's technique has been developed and has two major advantages:

1. By tightly packing the uterine cavity with source capsules, a closer approximation of the sources to the tumor and a more evenly distributed radiation dose are obtained.
2. Tightly packing the uterine cavity can bring about stretching of the walls of the uterus and can provide for a deeper dose within the myometrium (Fig. 4.27).

The number of sources depends upon the size of uterus. The second insertion will usually result in a lower number of capsules being inserted due to shrinkage of the uterus after the first insertion. It is given by two packings of 15–36 h each with Heyman's capsules at intervals of 2–3 weeks, each capsule being loaded with 8–10 mg ^{226}Ra. Two vaginal ovoids are also used on the first packing. A total dose of 30 Gy at a depth of 1.5 cm to the endometrial surface is obtained.

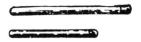

Intrauterine Applicators with different sizes

Supporters of vaginal applicators
(might be loaded with 2-5 radiation units)

Radiation unit

Vaginal applicator loaded with 4 radiation units

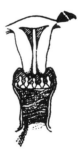

Schematic diagram in a combined intrauterine
and vaginal application

Fig. 4.26. Beijing method for Intracavitary Radiation

4.3.2.1.4 Afterloading

A major problem of intracavitary irradiation is that of exposure of medical staff
to irradiation. With the afterloading system, the empty source carrier is inserted
into the treatment position within the patient and held there with a suitable

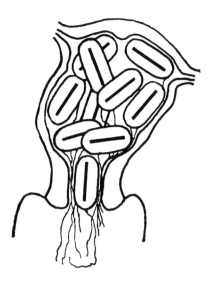

Fig. 4.27. Heyman uterine packing system. Tightly packing the uterine cavity with Heyman capsules

clamping system. Then the radioactive sources are moved from storage into the carrier in the patient automatically. With the availability of an afterloading device, a full radiation protective system may be provided. In rapid dose afterloading intracavitary radiotherapy with strong radioactive sources in the applicators utilizing very short treatment times, new complicated radiobiologic problems have been introduced in intracavitary radiation. But this technique is still under development and more knowledge and experience is needed to evaluate this type of treatment as far as immediate results and late radiation injuries are concerned. The Buchler remote afterloading device has been used in the Cancer Institute Hospital, Beijing. The Buchler remote afterloading device consists of a single, almost pinpoint, source, for short irradiation with a high dose, which oscillates in the applicator. The applicator consists of a probe made of stainless steel with a diameter of 8 mm. During the process of treatment, the source movement is checked and recorded via a measuring probe and at the same time continuous monitoring of the radiation level in the rectum and the bladder is performed via separate dosemeter probes in these organs. A program disk is shaped so as to determine the dose distribution and control the oscillating source. The most frequently used isodose curves can be reproduced with only eight disks. No. 8 and No. 9 program disks can produce a suitable dose distribution for treatment in endometrial carcinoma (Fig. 4.28).

4.3.2.2 Intracavitary Radiation

4.3.2.2.1 Preoperative Intracavitary Radiation

For intracavitary insertions, it is a common practice to use the tandem or to pack the uterine cavity with Heyman's capsules. With a small uterine cavity, two

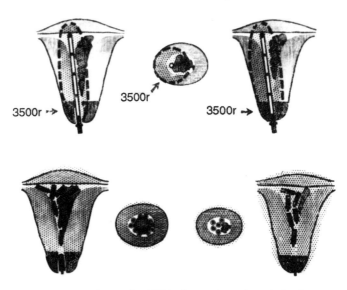

Fig. 4.28. *Upper*, a tandem in the uterine cavity. With the tandem, there is inadequate irradiation to the tumor and myometrium in the first insertion (*left*) and again in the second insertion (*right*); In contrast, with Heyman's capsules, the tumor is surrounded by radium sources (*lower left*) and, having shrunk considerably between the two insertions, the serosal surface receives a more uniform dose (*lower right*). (Adapted from Chau 1962, p. 244)

Heyman-type packings or tandem applications together with one application of vaginal ovoids 2–3 weeks apart to give a total dose of 35 Gy or 2000–3000 mg h. With an enlarged uterus (>8 cm), the Heyman-type packings should be used.

The interval between completion of radiotherapy and hysterectomy is based on the reactive degree of tissues in the pelvis to radiation. The immediate radiation reactions appear to reach the peak of reactions after 2 weeks and then decrease gradually. About 6 weeks later, the occlusion of blood vessels and fibrosis appeared; and the outline of tissues tended to be clear and the opportunity for infection decreased. The recommended interval from radiation to hysterectomy varies from immediately to 6 weeks.

Preoperative intracavitary radiation using the afterloading technique has been used in the Cancer Institute Hospital, Beijing. The applicator of the Buchler remote afterloading device is equipped with ^{192}Ir (iridium-192). A dose of 10–20 Gy has been given to point A, which is one-third or one-half the doses for primary radiotherapy. The dose from intracavitary radiation is calculated to be 10–20 Gy at point F, i.e., 2 cm lateral to the middle line at fundus level, which is similar to that at point A. The recommended interval from radiation to hysterectomy could be 7–10 days in this hospital.

4.3.2.2.2 Postoperative Intravaginal Radiation

Postoperative intravaginal radiation should be administered to the patients who have cervical involvement and carcinoma at the vaginal cutting edges in the hysterectomy specimen and given 2–4 weeks after hysterectomy.

4.3.2.2.3 Primary Intracavitary Radiation

Primary intracavitary radiation may be used for the patients who have contraindications for surgery or refuse to be given an operation. ^{226}Ra or ^{137}Cs may be used as a radiation source. The patient with a small or normal-sized uterine cavity is treated with tandem and vaginal ovoids, which are usually given in four to five or seven to eight sittings each of 20–22 h duration separated by 7 days. The total radiation dose in 6000 to 10 000 mgh, while the uterine dose should be 3000–4000 mgh. The interval between the sittings also depends upon the tumor regression and the patient's general condition. In the patient with a large uterus, Heyman packings may be used, which may be followed by tandem application . The total dose should be 60 Gy at 1.5 cm from the surface of the radiation source and the vaginal dose should be 1500–3000 mgh.

The rapid dose remote afterloading technique is also used in the primary intracavitary radiation in the Cancer Institute Hospital, Beijing. The total dose is calculated to be 40 Gy at point F in four fractions separated by 7 days.

4.3.2.3 Preoperative Intracavitary or Postoperative Intravaginal Irradiation as an Adjunct to Surgery

In a review of the literature, it appears that vaginal recurrence rates are reduced when surgery is supplemented with preoperative intracavitary or postoperative intravaginal irradiation (Table 4.8). However, there is no evidence that the overall survival is improved (Graham 1971; Jones 1975; McCabe and Sagerman 1979; Piver 1980).

Advantages and disadvantages have been claimed for preoperative intra-uterine or postoperative intravaginal irradiation. Even both of them can reduce the vaginal recurrence rates. Preoperative intracavitary irradiation offers the following advantages and disadvantages.

The advantages are (a) lowering of the vaginal recurrence rate, (b) shrinkage of the primary tumor making it more operable, and (c) reduction of vascular dissemination when operating.

The disadvantages are: (a) delayed definite treatment, (b) difficulty in making assessment of myometrial invasion, and (c) higher radiation complication rates making operation difficult.

Postoperative intravaginal irradiation offers the following advantages and disadvantages. The advantages are: (a) lowering of the vaginal recurrence rate,

Table 4.8. Vaginal recurrences following therapy: hysterectomy alone versus hysterectomy and radiation

| Series | Year | Vaginal recurrence | | | |
		S (%)	S + PreIUR (%)	S + PostIVR (%)	S + PostExR ± PostIVR (%)
Rutledge et al.	1958	20.0	1.5	–	–
Dobbie	1953	5.5	0	1.8	–
Graham	1971	12.0	3	–	–
Beiler et al.	1972	12.0	1.6	–	–
Onsrud et al.	1976	–	–	4.6	2.1
Joslin et al.	1977	–	–	3.6	3.0
Joslin	1985	–	–	1.5	–

S, surgery; PreIUR, preoperative intrauterine radiation; PostIVR, postoperative intravaginal radiation; PostExR, postoperative external radiation.

(b) definite primary management without delay, and (c) reduction of suburethral recurrence.

The disadvantage is that morbidity may be high, such as vaginal stenosis, recurrent proctitis, and cystitis.

In view of the above discussion, it is advisable to use preoperative intracavitary or postoperative intravaginal irradiation as an adjunctive therapy depending on the individual treatment schedule. The indication of adjunctive radiation should strictly be controlled in the clinical management of endometrial carcinoma.

4.3.2.4 Comments on Preoperative Radiation Therapy

4.3.2.4.1 Rationale for the Use of Preoperative Radiation Therapy

The rationale for the use of preoperative radiation therapy has been discussed and the following five theoretical advantages have been proposed (Rutledge et al. 1958; Truskett and Constable 1968; Sall et al. 1970; Jones 1975).

1. Radiation sterilizes a certain proportion of malignancies.
2. A bulky soft uterus shrinks, making subsequent operations easier.
3. Metastatic channels are obliterated, reducing the possibility of retrograde spread.
4. Vault recurrences are reduced.
5. The 5-year survival is improved.

Randall and Goddard (1956), Silverberg and DeGiorgi (1974), and Nahhas et al. (1984) indicated that preoperative radiation therapy would not be very efficient in removing all neoplastic tissues from the uterus especially when the tissue was in the myometrium. The basic question remains of whether the irradiated neoplastic cells are viable and able to implant, metastasize, and continue to grow. Most authors agree that although the irradiated neoplastic cells can be viable they would not be capable of implanting if spread occurred at the time of operation. They support the concept of a lower incidence of vaginal vault recurrence in patients treated with preoperative radiation plus surgery.

4.3.2.4.2 General Impression of Preoperative Radiation Therapy

1. Residual carcinoma is present in 16%–75% of uteri removed following radiation therapy (Gusberg and Yannopoulos 1964; Sall et al. 1970).
2. The incidence of residual tumor in the irradiated uterus is inversely proportional to the time interval between radiation therapy and hysterectomy (Boronow 1969; Silverberg and DeGiorgi 1974).
3. Even though residual tumor can be readily identified and is morphologically intact and similar to the preoperative histology, the cells are radiobiologically damaged and are incapable of implantation (Suit and Shalek 1963; Suit and Gallager 1964).

The correlation between residual carcinoma in the irradiated uteri and prognosis has been the subject of controversy. Taylor and Becker (1947) and Randall and Goddard (1956) were among the first authors to associate a poor prognosis with the presence of residual disease in the uterus treated with preoperative radiation. Silverberg and DeGiorgi (1974) reported that, in 76 patients treated with preoperative irradiation, only 29% had no tumor at the time of hysterectomy and the 5-year survival rate in this group was 80%; the majority of patients had residual disease and the 5-year survival rate was reduced to 60%. Kjellgren and Magnusson (1970) and Surwit et al. (1981) concluded that the absence of tumor in the surgical specimen of their patients with stage I poorly differentiated tumors who received preoperative radium correlated well with survival. Preoperative intracavitary radiation therapy for these patients was recommended. No correlation between residual disease and survival was reported by Sala and Del Regato (1961) Badib et al. (1969), Marcial et al. (1969), Vongtama et al. (1970), and Nahhas et al. (1980).

4.3.2.4.3 Factors Affecting the Presence of Residual Carcinoma

At present, it is also unclear whether the behavior of residual tumor following only intracavitary brachytherapy is different from the residual tumor following external radiation therapy. The factors affecting the presence of residual carcinoma from the literature have been summarized as follows:

1. Kadar et al. (1982) concluded that the frequency of residual tumor found at the time of hysterectomy was similar regardless of the therapeutic modality

utilized: external pelvic irradiation with or without intracavitary therapy. This is consistent with the results obtained by Nahhas et al. (1984). In their series, 71% of patients with external radiation therapy had residual carcinoma compared with 68% of patients with combination therapy.

2. The histology of the original tumor has been considered a factor affecting the presence of residual carcinoma. In one study, 40% of the uteri containing well-differentiated adenocarcinoma were sterilized with preoperative irradiation as compared with only 12% of poorly differentiated tumors (Silverberg and DeGiorgi 1974). Nahhas et al. (1984) reported that 37% of the uteri which contained well-differentiated adenocarcinoma had no residual tumor compared with 21% of those with less-differentiated lesions (grades II, III), but this difference was not statistically significant.

3. The time interval between completion of radiation therapy and removal of the uterus has been accepted as a variable that may influence the incidence of residual tumor. Boronow (1969) showed no significant difference in survival related to the radium-hysterectomy interval when the uterus was removed from 0 to 10 weeks following completion of radiation therapy. Even though 90% of the uteri removed within 5 weeks may show a residual tumor as compared with only 45% removed between 5 and 10 weeks following completion of therapy, there is no evidence that delay in performing hysterectomy improves survival (Silverberg and DeGorgi 1974). It can be postulated that, given enough time, the irradiated cells will spontaneously disappear and will have no appreciable effect on the recurrence rate and on survival.

4. The depth of myometrial invasion by tumor prior to radiation therapy has also been considered as a variable that can affect residual carcinoma. Silverberg and DeGiorgi (1974) and Surwit et al. (1981) concluded that the major prognostic indicator was the presence of residual tumor invading the myometrium. Tumor within the myometrium was difficult to eradicate with radiation therapy, which did not change the morphologic appearance of the carcinoma in the myometrium, which remained histologically similar to the preradiation therapy curettings (Sall et al. 1970; Silverberg and DeGiorgi 1974; Nahhas et al. 1984). Even deep myometrial invasion by tumor in uterine specimens removed prior to radiation therapy is known to be a poor prognostic indicator as it remains unclear whether residual tumor within the myometrium following radiation therapy has similar significance. Frick et al. (1973) and Berman et al. (1982) showed that the depth of myometrial invasion was less valuable as a prognostic indicator in patients treated initially with radiation therapy.

4.3.2.4.4 Disadvantages of Preoperative Radiation Therapy

The disadvantages are:

1. Preoperative radiation therapy distorts the histopathologic picture of the tumor and makes any estimation of myometrial invasion difficult.

2. Before surgicopathologic staging, preoperative radiation therapy can only be given blindfold, because preoperative radiation therapy is confined within the pelvis but the extensive involvement of tumor out of the pelvis is usually found during operation.
3. It affects the components of tumor and makes measurement of receptor impossible.

As mentioned above, preoperative radiation therapy has not been used routinely.

4.3.2.4.5 Indications for Preoperative Intracavitary Radiation Therapy

1. Overt stage II endometrial carcinoma should preferably be treated with preoperative intracavitary radiation therapy. It means preoperative radiotherapy may be used for those stage II patients diagnosed on speculum examination.
2. It is advisable in all grade III lesions.
3. For enlarged and soft uterus, preoperative intracavitary radiation therapy can shrink the primary tumor and reduce the uterine volume, making operation easier and reducing dissemination of cancer at hysterectomy.

4.3.3 External Beam Therapy

4.3.3.1 Preoperative External Beam Therapy

In 1941, Wintz first reported the effect of preoperative external beam therapy in combination with surgery in the treatment of endometrial carcinoma. His results showed approximately a 69% 5-year survival. In 1963, Lampe used deep X-ray therapy to deliver 40 Gy in 3–4 weeks in 121 patients with stage I disease followed by a hysterectomy and bilateral salpingo-oophorectomy (BSO) 6 weeks later. He reported a 90% 5-year survival. Salazar et al. (1978) studied preoperative external beam therapy according to uterine size. For a small uterus, a tandem and ovoids were used to deliver 30 Gy to the Manchester point A, followed by 50 Gy to the central pelvis and 45 Gy to the pelvic side wall with supervoltage therapy. For a large uterus, Heyman's capsules were used to deliver 40 Gy at 1 cm into the myometrium and external therapy as previously. Of the 155 cases, surgical complications occurred in 10% and there were 5% chronic radiation problems. At 5 years 82% were alive without evidence of disease. On reviewing the literature, Salazar reported 87% survival in 362 cases. This is significantly better ($P < 0.05$) than that of patients with initial surgery (80%) or preoperative intracavitary therapy (80%). Gagnon et al. (1979) reported on 24 stage II patients receiving preoperative external beam therapy. A dose of 45–50 Gy was given. Surgery performed 4–5 weeks later in 23 cases of these patients revealed local residual disease in 14 of them (61%), suggesting, for the dose given, that external beam therapy alone will not cure extensive local disease. The adjusted survival rate at 5 years was estimated to be 81%. By 5 years, of the four recurrences, one was vaginal metastasis, one pulmonary metastasis, one liver metastasis, and the last one abdominal metastasis. Ritcher et al. (1981) reported a 95% 5-year survival in 161 patients with stage I disease, who had preoperative external beam radiotherapy. The dose delivered ranged from 10.5 to 67 Gy at a rate of 1.8–2.0 Gy/day, most patients receiving 35 Gy. This was followed 1–2 weeks later by operation, and very few complications were encountered. Shimm et al. (1986) recommended that patients with FIGO stage I, grade III adenocarcinoma of the endometrium receive external pelvic radiation of 10 Gy in four fractions followed by operation within a week. The operation included hysterectomy and BSO, sampling the paraaortic lymph nodes, as well as pelvic and peritoneal washings. In his series of 68 FIGO stage I patients treated with this protocol, an 80% probability of 5-year disease-free survival for patients with grade III carcinoma was observed.

To date, this form of therapy has not been used very often as the advantages of preoperative external radiation are outweighed by its disadvantages. Definite treatment is delayed, complication rates are high, and there is no evidence that the reduction rate of vaginal recurrence is lower than that with preoperative intracavitary radiation, so preoperative external beam therapy alone can only be used in the following conditions:

1. The uterine cavity is so large that it cannot be packed tightly with Heyman capsules.
2. For advanced disease, it shrinks the primary tumor and involves lymph nodes within the pelvis, making operation easier.

The recommended interval from radiation to hysterectomy varies from 4 to 6 weeks. An opposing field technique may be used and the entire dose given with an 8 MV linear accelerator. By using two opposing fields with a lead shielding block measuring $18 \times 15 cm^2$, which covers the lymph node areas of the pelvis, a lead shield is placed over the central part of the pelvis. This shield is 15 cm long and 4–5 cm wide. Lead shields of different designs are also used. The external radiation of the pelvis should also be given a rhombic field, measuring 10 $\times$ 10 cm^2. A daily tumor dose of 2 Gy 5 days a week may be given to most patients. A homogenous dose throughout the pelvis of 30 Gy may be given over 4 weeks. Full preoperative pelvic external irradiation is advisable in lesions affecting the parametrium and having severe bleeding.

4.3.3.2 Postoperative External Beam Therapy

During the 1940s, interest focussed on the use of postoperative irradiation. Masson and Gregg (1940) reported postoperative external X-ray therapy to improve the survival of those patients who were found to have no satisfactory reaction to other modalities of therapy. In 1977, Joslin et al. reported the results of using postoperative intravaginal and external beam therapy. A prescribed tumor dose of 35 Gy delivered in 15 fractions over 21 days followed by intravaginal treatment of 20 Gy in four fractions over 3 days was given. The latter has been reduced to 16 Gy in four fractions and then to 12 Gy also in four fractions. The results indicate that a reduction in pelvic recurrence occurred, the overall 5-year survival being 91%. The use of external beam therapy is based on the surgicopathologic examination and complications do not seem very high. Postoperative external beam therapy has been widely used, the aim of which is to (a) cure involved lymph nodes and metastatic cancer foci within and above the pelvis, which are found during operation and cannot be resected, and (b) depending upon pathologic evaluation of the operative specimen, some prognostic factors are to be found such as grade III lesions, deeper myometrial infiltration, lesions affecting the cervix, and isthmus of the uterus, microscopic adnexal involvement, and adenosquamous or clear cell carcinoma.

In general, full pelvic external radiation may be used. Two opposing fields measuring 18×15 cm^2 are used, which cover the lymph node area of the pelvis and vagina. A homogeneous dose throughout the pelvis of 40–50 Gy may be given over 4–5 weeks. A smaller sized field should be constructed for the paraaortic lymph node area if paraaortic lymph node metastases are present. In the Cancer Institute Hospital, Beijing, postoperative external beam therapy has become popular. The entire dose is given by 8-MV linear accelerator and an opposing field technique may be used. By using two parallel-opposing fields measuring 17×14 cm^2 or 18×15 cm^2, the entire tumor dose throughout the pelvis of 40–45 Gy is given in 5–6 weeks.

4.3.3.3 External Beam Therapy Alone

External beam therapy alone should be reserved for advanced disease (stages III, IV) and stage I and II disease only if operation and internal radiation are contraindicated.

4.3.3.3.1 Primary Full Pelvic External Beam Irradiation

Anterior and posterior parallel opposed fields of 15×15 cm^2 or a rhombic field of 10×10 cm^2 are used. A homogeneous dose of 50–60 Gy is given to the whole pelvis over 5–6 weeks. During the external irradiation, if the tumor appears to diminish and if it is technically possible to insert carriers into the uterus, some form of intracavitary treatment may be followed. Two opposing fields with lead shielding block irradiation can be used instead of full pelvic external beam irradiation. The entire dose is calculated to be approximately 40–45 Gy. The vagina must be covered in order to prevent vaginal recurrence.

4.3.3.3.2 Moving Strip Whole Abdomen Radiation

This was first developed by Paterson (1948) and later by Delclos et al. (1963) for telecobalt therapy and more recently by Dembo et al. (1979). This technique delivers a high radiologically effective dose to the abdomen which has been used for patients with extensive abdominal and pelvic metastases. A total abdominal dose of 26–28 Gy in 12 fractions over 30–40 days is normally given.

These fields are set up to cover the abdomen from the dome of the diaphragm to the pelvic floor. The liver and kidneys are carefully protected from radiation. The aim of the strip field is to provide a better therapeutic ratio by arranging treatment in a series of strips 2.5 cm wide each. Parallel opposed strips are treated daily and the number of strips treated increases by one width every 2 days. Once a total width of 10 cm is reached, the process is moved up 2.5 cm and the first strip is left off. Treatment starts from the pelvic floor level following the initial treatment to the dome of the diaphragm.

4.4 Hormonal Treatment

Endometrial carcinoma is one of the hormone-dependent tumors and can, therefore, respond to the antagonistic influences of progestogens and antiestrogens. In 1951, Kelley observed regression in two of three patients with endometrial carcinoma treated with progesterone. In 1961, Kelley and Baker of Harvard University, United States, first reported a 37% objective response to progestogens in metastatic endometrial carcinoma. Since then various progestogens have been tried for the treatment of advanced or recurrent endometrial carcinoma (Varga and Henriksen 1961; Wentz 1964, 1974, Smith et al. 1966; Malkasian et al. 1971; Geisler 1973; Wait 1973; Reifenstein 1974; Kohorn 1976). More recently, the hormone dependency and hormone responsiveness of gynecologic malignancies, which originated on theoretical and experimental grounds, have been based on the data provided by steroid receptor determination. Recent studies on the steroid receptor content of endometrial carcinoma provide more effective means of predicting response.

4.4.1 Progestogens

4.4.1.1 Mechanism

The effect of progestogens on endometrial carcinoma has demonstrated a decrease in the atypicality and pleomorphism of the glands and a decrease in epithelial metaplasia. The cytoplasm became more granular and eosinophilic, and secretory vacuoles appeared. Eventually the carcinoma was replaced by endometrial hyperplasia or by endometrial atrophy (Anderson 1965; Kistner et al. 1965; Kohorn 1976; Anderson 1972).

4.4.1.1.1 Cytobiologic Research

Progestogens affect the tumor directly and can inhibit the growth of human endometrial carcinoma cell lines in vitro (Reel 1976; Satya-swaroop et al. 1980). This growth inhibition is characterized by the normalization of nuclear morphology, a significant fall in DNA content and a decrease in polyploidy (Reel 1976). This growth inhibition is dose dependent (Reel 1976; Ishiwata et al. 1977; Satyaswaroop et al. 1980). Medroxyprogesterone acetate (MPA), at a concentration of 20 μg/ml, has been found to inhibit mitosis in more than 85% of endometrial carcinoma cell cultures. Progestogens induce a rapid and significant fall of cytosol ER (ERc) content in the cancer cells, inhibiting DNA synthesis (Reel 1976; Gurpide and Tseng 1977; Tseng et al. 1977; Janne 1979; Martin et al. 1979; Prodi et al. 1980; Vihko et al. 1980). The rapid changes in ERc levels suggest unmasking of receptors, rather than synthesis and degradation, which may be related to the cell cycle (Gurpide 1981). Progestogens also reduce the cytosol PR (PRc) content in endometrial carcinoma and the reasons for PRc reduction involve nuclear translocation and nonreplenishment of the receptor (Martin et al. 1979). During the long-term progestational treatment, PRc disappearance may affect the treatment results of progestogens (Reel 1976; Ishiwata et al. 1977; Janne 1979; Martin et al. 1979; Prodi et al. 1980; Satyaswaroop et al. 1980; Vihko et al. 1980; Barni et al. 1981). Bonte (1984) presented data showing the patients with endometrial adenocarcinoma were treated with 150 mg 1 day medroxyprogesterone, and ER and PR contents were observed during treatment. Of the ER-positive adenocarcinomas, 75% showed a decrease in receptor content, while tumors totally devoid of ER revealed no change at all. But the reduction of PR content was observed in all cases of endometrial carcinoma, which does not seem related to original PR content but is caused by exhaustion of the cytosol reserve.

4.4.1.1.2 Histologic Research

Microscopic Manifestation
The histologic response of the endometrial carcinoma was generally characterized by Bonte (1985): (a) enhanced secretory activity, with formation of subnuclear vacuoles; (b) transformation of pseudostratified cells to active monolayered glands (c) marked epithelial metaplasia of some glandular structures, especially in adenoacanthomatous tumors, (d) pseudodecidualization of the stroma and (e) atrophy of the epithelium and fibrosis of the stroma, leading to the break-down of the tumor substance.

Holincka and Gurpide (1980) pointed out that a progestational response may appear in the superficial adenocarcinoma, but infiltrating adenocarcinoma in the myometrium does not reveal any subnuclear vacuolization.

Histochemical Change
There is substantial accumulation of glycogen, glyco-proteins, and mucopolysaccharides in the cytoplasm.

Ultrastructural Response
There is secretory conversion, decrease in length of microvilli, and loss of cilia (Ferenczy 1977).

4.4.1.1.3 Biochemical Research

Progestogen induces the enzyme 17-β-hydroxysteroid dehydrogenase (17-β-DH). This enzyme catalyzes the conversion of estradiol (E_2) to estrone (E_1) and reduces the level of E_2 in the cell (Gurpide 1979). During the high-dose progestogen administration, a change in the unsaturated 2-position fatty acids of serum lecithin was seen. Moreover, an increase in the relative amount of linoleic acid was paralleled by a decrease in arachidonic acid. After the high-dose administration, a redistribution in the 1-position saturated fatty acids of serum lecithin was seen. Accordingly, the relative content of palmitic acid increased concomitantly with a decrease in stearic acid (Enk et al. 1985). Changes in the fatty acid composition of serum phospholipids are paralleled by changes in the phospholipids of the cell membrane. Recent experimental data show that high-dose MPA induces structural changes in the lipid bilayer of the cell membrane and produces the antitumor activity (Bojar et al. 1983). This activity may appear within the first 3 months of treatment and remained constant thereafter.

4.4.1.1.4 Endocrinologic Research

Vaginal Smear Cytology
A shift of the vaginal smear to atrophy is the typical change in progestogen treatment, especially for the patients with hormone-responsive adenocarcinoma.

Serum Hormonal Levels
Administration of 1 g medroxyprogesterone weekly induces no significant changes in estradiol (E_2) and estrone (E_1) plasma concentrations. There are no statistically significant changes in steroid hormone plasma levels under medium-dosed medroxyprogesterone administration (Vesterinen et al. 1981). During the medroxyprogesterone treatment, the fall in follicle-stimulating (FSH) plasma levels is statistically significant for the whole patient group but the fall in

luteinizing hormone (LH) is statistically significant for the responsive group only (Vesterinen et al. 1981).

4.4.1.2 Pharmacokinetics of Progestogens

The aim of pharmacokinetic research is how to reach the effective drug levels soon and to maintain them until progression of the disease. After single intramuscular administration, the MPA plasma levels are very low, about 1 ng/ml for each 100-mg dose and decreasing slowly. The elimination, $t_{1/2}$, from the plasma takes about 6 weeks. Owing to the slow and long-lasting absorption from the injection sites, every repeated dose treatment at regular intervals will result in an extensive accumulation of drug plasma levels until a steady-state situation which will be reached only after 6–8 months of treatment. When the intramuscular therapy is discontinued, the drug levels will decrease very slowly and a maintenance therapy of 1 g/week is sufficient to maintain indefinitely the high MPA plasma levels achieved with the loading phase (Salimtschik et al. 1980; Tamassia et al. 1982). After a single oral administration, peak plasma MPA levels much higher than those achieved after comparable intramuscular doses are rapidly reached, but elimination is relatively rapid with a plasma $t_{1/2}$ of about 2 days (Salimtschik et al. 1980). During the first 10 days of treatment, there is a building-up phase of drug plasma levels followed by a steady-state situation where MPA plasma levels are linearly related to the daily dose administration (about 10 ng/ml for each 100-mg oral daily dose). Any reduction in the dose or discontinuation of treatment will result in a rapid, proportional decrease in MPA levels within 10 days (Tamassia et al. 1982). Tamassia (1986) concluded that a pharmacokinetically rational dose schedule of intramuscular MPA should be based on a loading phase of daily injections for 2–4 weeks followed by a maintenance treatment with weekly injections. Even oral and intramuscular MPA are not equivalent. It is possible to design and adopt dose schedules for both routes of administration which are equipotential in terms of MPA plasma level profile.

Sall et al. (1979) reported their data to compare the serum medroxyprogesterone concentrations administered through the oral and intramuscular routes. The oral group received 50 mg three times a day, and the intramuscular group received 300 mg weekly for at least 2 months. Serum levels were evaluated daily at 0, 2, 4, 6, 8, 10, and 12 h after administration for the 1st week and weekly thereafter for 8 weeks. The mean serum levels of medroxyprogesterone in the oral group were consistently higher than the corresponding mean levels of the intramuscular group. This shows that the measurements for the oral group were statistically higher than those for the intramuscular group if medroxyprogesterone is given orally at suitable intervals. Tamassia (1986) reported their pharmacokinetic data based on medroxyprogesterone plasma level determinations. The same plasma levels of medroxyprogesterone could be achieved through either the oral or the intramuscular route (Table 4.9).

Table 4.9. Equipotent oral and intramuscular MPA dose schedules. (Adapted from Tamassia 1986)

Oral MPA daily doses (mg)	Plasma levels (mean) (ng/ml)	Intramuscular MPA	
		Loading (cumulative/ 4 weeks) (g)	Maintenance (mg/week)
250	≃25	3	250
500	≃50	6	500
1000	≃100	12–14	1000
1500	≃150	20	1500

Medium-dose medroxyprogesterone administration which may give plasma concentrations in excess of the 90 ng/ml medroxyprogesterone threshold measured by radioimmunoassay achieves an excellent objective remission rate. The plasma concentrations easily exceed the 90-ng/ml level after the 1st week of daily oral medroxyprogesterone at a dose of 150 mg and after the 5th week of weekly intramuscular injection at a dose of 1 g medroxyprogesterone (Bonte 1985). The various types of progestogen and administration routes are shown in Table 4.10.

4.4.1.3 Clinical Data

Kelley and Baker (1961) first reported a 37% objective response to progestogens in the metastatic endometrial carcinoma. Since then progestogen therapy has been recommended for advanced metastatic or recurrent disease. The best response is expected in well-differentiated lesions ranging from 30% to 35% (Bonte and Kohorn 1978, Bonte 1980; Piver et al. 1980). The response to progestogens may be related to (a) the type and route of administration of the progestational compound and (b) the response of the tumor to the drug. The response of the tumor is determined by the type of progestogen, the plasma levels, and the characteristics of the tumor such as the degree of differentiation, the duration of recurrence, the receptor content, and recurrent, metastatic locations. The plasma progestogen concentrations are related to the dose, administration route, and administration schedule. According to the present data, no direct dose-response relationship in the progestational treatment of endometrial carcinoma could be found. However, the mean medroxyprogesterone bioavailability is dose dependent with small day-to-day intraindividual but rather high interindividual variations (Laatikainen et al. 1979; Pannutti 1981).

Table 4.10. Progestational agents and their usage in endometrial carcinoma

Drug	Route	Schedule
Derivatives of 17α-hydroxyprogesterone		
17α-Hydroxyprogesterone caproate	i.m.	500 mg qd for 2 months, then 500 mg qod for 6 months, then 500 mg/week
Medroxyprogesterone	i.m.	100 mg qd for 10 days, then 200 mg 3 times a week 10 times, then 100–200 mg/week
Megestrol	Oral	40–80 mg qd
Chloromedinone	Oral	20–40 mg qd
Medroxyprogesterone acetate (MPA)	Oral	150 mg qd or 50–100 mg qd
Derivatives of 19 normethyltesto-sterone		
Nogestrol	Oral	10–20 mg qd

The studies on MPA administration show that medium-dose MPA administration, inducing plasma concentrations exceeding 90 ng/ml, achieves an excellent objective remission rate. Plasma concentrations exceed the 90 ng/ml level after the 1st week of daily oral 150 mg provera administration and after the 5th week of weekly intramuscular 1 g depo provera. Plasma LH levels and vaginal smear may be used for monitoring the response of the adenocarcinoma. Hormone sensitivity to oral MPA treatment becomes apparent within 10 days by an abrupt fall of plasma LH levels, by an elevation of plasma MPA levels beyond 90 ng/ml, and by a sudden change toward atrophy in the vaginal smear (Bonte 1979).

Based on individual reports, a comparison of the mean objective remission rates for the most frequently used progestational compounds is as follows: progesterone, 56%; medroxyprogesterone acetate, 35%–57%; megestrol, 33%–41%; megestrone, 21%–34%; and hydroxyprogesterone caproate, 18% –33% (Bonte 1979; Caffier et al. 1982).

The practical advantage of medroxyprogesterone for oral cancer therapy becomes evident because of the difficulties of intramuscular injection of progesterone for a long period. Bonte (1980) reported a series of 115 patients treated orally with 150 mg/day medroxyprogesterone. The objective remission rate was 51%. The average duration of remissions was 11 months and the duration of survival reached 20 moths.

Progestogens produce in the patient a sensation of well-being by the relief of pain, improved appetite, and gain in weight. The incidence of side effects of nausea, vomiting, and fluid retention could be very low, and phlebitis, cerebrovascular disease, and pulmonary embolism might occasionally be observed.

There is still controversy on the results of progestogens in the treatment of endometrial carcinoma in the literature. Thigpen et al. (1985) reported the studies conducted by the Gynecologic Oncology Group Study of the United States. A total of 413 patients with recurrent or advanced endometrial carcinoma were treated with MPA, 50 mg orally three times/day. The median period of treatment was 3 months, ranging from 1 to 43 months. The overall objective response rate of 14% was lower than that reported in the earlier literature. Progestins appear to be less active than previously expected in the treatment of endometrial carcinoma. Bokhman et al. (1981) presented the results of pre-operative use of oxyprogesterone caproate (OPC) in 398 patients with primary endometrial carcinoma. OPC was injected daily at a dose of 500 mg. Each patient received from 10.0 to 16.0 g OPC before operation. Positive effects of hormone therapy were observed in 75.8% of cases (44 out of 58 patients). In 14 out of 58 patients a complete regression of the tumor took place. It shows that the cure of endometrial carcinoma as a result of OPC treatment without surgical and irradiative intervention is possible. The complete regression of the tumor may be attained in a greater number of patients when the duration of OPC treatment and its course dosage are increased. Moazzami et al. (1983) reported that 59 patients with stage I endometrial carcinoma were treated with total abdominal hysterectomy (TAH), BSO, followed by gestronal hexanoate for 3 months and then MPA orally for a prolonged period. There were no vaginal recurrences in 7 years. In addition, the absence of any complications associated with progestogen administration compared favorably with the reported incidence of complications after adjuvant radiotherapy. But this study cannot be regarded as definite proof that progestogens can replace radiotherapy as an adjunct to surgery in the treatment of stage I endometrial carcinoma. Lewis et al. (1974) reported that depoprovera and placebo given over 14 weeks were randomly assigned in such a way that 285 patients received hormone and 287 served as controls. The option of surgery alone or surgery plus irradiation was permitted to all patients. Survival analysis at 4 years indicated no significant contribution to results by the adjuvant hormone therapy.

Hormone treatment may be used for young patients with confined disease in the uterus, but the pathogenetic characteristics of the organism which promote the development of endometrial cancer may persist after the completion of hormone treatment and may induce recurrence of the disease. It is necessary to strive to remove anovulation and obesity and to compensate hyperlipidemia and glucose intolerance, in order to prevent not only the recurrence of endometrial carcinoma but also the development of hormone-dependent multiple primary tumors (cancers of the breast and colon) (Annegers and Malkasian 1981). Bokhman et al. (1985) presented a hormone treatment schedule. Hydroxy-progesterone caproate (HPC) was administered intramuscularly at the dose of 500 mg/day. The sensitivity of the tumor to HPC was checked every week through cytologic examination of the endometrial aspirations. The first part of the treatment lasted 3 months, after which biopsy of the endometrium was carried out. If histologic examination showed adenocarcinoma after this period of treatment, surgery was performed. In cases where no tumor elements were revealed in the specimen obtained from the second biopsy, the treatment was continued for another 3 months. A dose of 500 mg HPC was given intramuscularly twice a week. A 6-month antiestrogen treatment usually results in endometrial atrophy and amenorrhea. During the second part of the treatment, an artificial cycle was introduced with the administration of combined steroid contraceptives for three to four cycles. The next step was the restoration of ovulation with clomiphene citrate followed by chorionic gonadotrophins. It is necessary to emphasize that hormone therapy as a separate method treatment of endometrial carcinoma is at present at the pilot investigation stage.

4.4.2 Antiestrogens

4.4.2.1 Mechanism

The synthetic nonsteroid antiestrogens of a series of triphenylethylenes have estroantiestrogenic activity. One of these compounds, tamoxifen (the *trans* isomer of 1-(p-dimethylaminoethoxyphenyl)-1,2-diphenylbut-1-ene) (TAM), has been used for the treatment of endometrial carcinoma.

4.4.2.1.1 Cytobiologic Research

Tamoxifen has been shown to increase progesterone receptor (PR) concentration in the rodent uterus, while it counteracts estrogen-induced uterine growth (Jordan and Dix 1978). TAM behaves as a pure antiestrogen in the chick oviduct as far as growth, ovalbumin synthesis, or PR concentration are concerned (Sutherland et al. 1977).

Tamoxifen can attack the adenocarcinomatous cells by direct inhibition of mitosis. If TAM (1–2 µg/ml) is added to the medium and measured by means of tritiated thymidine incorporation, the mitotic index of endometrial adenocarcinoma in organotypic culture is markedly reduced in more than 40% of the cultures (Bonte 1981). TAM can inhibit the binding of estradiol to the cytosol estrogen receptor, reduce the concentration of these receptors, and interfere with the replenishment of the cytosol estrogen receptor (ER) in the endometrial cells. TAM may stimulate progesterone receptor synthesis. Similar action on endometrial carcinoma may be exerted by TAM (Robel et al. 1978; Mortel et al. 1981). The steroid receptor variations induced by TAM seem to depend on the original receptor concentration in the tumor cells. In all endometrial adenocarcinomas with a high ER content, daily 40-mg TAM administration induces an ER decrease after 7 days; in endometrial adenocarcinomas with low ER content, however, TAM provokes an ER increase, and in endometrial adenocarcinomas without ER, TAM produces either no change or an ER synthesis. TAM induces synthesis or an increase in PR in 71% of endometrial adenocarcinoma cells devoid of PR or with a low PR content, and TAM produces an increase in only 33% of high PR-containing endometrial adenocarcinomas (Bonte 1983).

4.4.2.1.2 Histologic Research

Microscopic Manifestation
At the normal dosage of TAM, 20 mg twice or three times a day, different histologic and histochemical transformations are produced according to tumor differentiation. The pseudostratified glands of the moderately differentiated adenocarcinoma are rapidly transformed into monolayered structures consisting of high cylindrical and, later on, even atrophic cells. Well-differentiated cancers develop atrophy and even necrosis. All responsive tumors are characterized by the decidualization of their stroma.

Histochemical Change
Tamoxifen sometimes induces glycogen with rare mucropolysaccharide accumulation (Bonte et al. 1981).

4.4.2.1.3 Endocrinologic Research

Vaginal Smear Cytology
Under short-term TAM treatment, the vaginal smear remains mostly estrogenic. Long-term TAM therapy induces a shift of the vaginal smear to a phase characteristic of a high or medium estrogenic stimulation in 60% of patients, and the vaginal smear remains unchanged in 35%. The cytologic change seems to occur irrespective of tumor response to TAM (Ferrazzi et al. 1977).

Serum Hormonal Levels
Tamoxifen provokes not only a fall in LH but also a fall in prolactin (Groom and Griffiths 1976) and a slight decrease in estradiol and estrone serum levels (Marchesoni et al. 1980; Bonte et al. 1981). In these postmenopausal women, the direct action of TAM on the normal ovary to stimulate estradiol release without intermediary gonadotropin stimulation is out of the question (Groom and Griffiths 1976).

4.4.2.2 Clinical Data

Tamoxifen at a daily dosage of 20–40 mg was administered orally in the first- and second-line treatment of metastatic or recurrent endometrial adenocarcinoma. Hald (1981) reported that an objective remission rate of 36% lasting from 8

to 45 months was achieved in his preliminary first-line treatment. A survey of approximately 50 patients with metastatic or recurrent endo-metrial adenocarcinoma treated with TAM at conventional dosage reveals an objective remission rate varying from 25% to 27% and a duration of 3 months up to more than 2 years (Bonte 1979; Swenerton et al. 1979; Broens et al. 1980; Swenerton 1980; Hald 1981; Kauppila and Fribert 1981; Quinn et al. 1981; Bonte 1983).
The clinical data of TAM may be summarized as follows:

1. There is a relationship between the dose of administration and the response of endometrial adenocarcinoma to TAM. Steady-state plasma concentrations ranging from 150 to 260 μg/ml are reached rather rapidly after regular daily administration of 20 mg TAM.
2. There is no proof that the response of endometrial adenocarcinoma to TAM is related to the cytosol estrogen receptor content of the tumor cells.
3. A close relationship is observed between the tumor response to medroxy-progesterone and that to TAM. The patients sensitive to second-line TAM therapy are those who previously responded to medroxyprogesterone (Swenerton et al. 1979; Swenerton 1980; Bonte et al. 1981) (Table 4.11).
4. The well-differentiated tumors with longer recurrent-free intervals are more likely to respond to TAM.
5. A dosage of 10–20 mg TAM twice per day orally is the conventional dosage.
6. With conventional doses, side effects of TAM are seldom observed and may disappear after reducing the dose or stopping the treatment. The potential side effects include nausea, vomiting, skin rashes, and vaginal bleeding. Hypercalcinemia and inhibition of bone marrow are seen in a few cases. Few patients are forced to stop the treatment because of the side effects.

4.4.3 Combination of Progestogens with Antiestrogens

In the treatment of endometrial carcinoma, progestogens and antiestrogens present different mechanisms which finally seem complementary to each other. A possible synergism between the simple antiestrogenic action of progestogens and the modulated, complex estroantiestrogenic activity of TAM has been established by long-term animal experiments. Moriel et al. (1984) concluded that sequential administration of TAM and progestin is superior to progestin alone in the treatment of receptor-positive endometrial adenocarcinoma. Progestogen treatment of advanced and recurrent endometrial carcinoma has been demonstrated to be rational. However, the response of endometrial carcinoma decreases after a long period of administration, as progestogens can finally extinguish their own efficiency by exhaustion of the PRc without the capacity for automatic replenishment. TAM stimulates PR synthesis in most tumors, increase the response of endometrial carcinoma to progestogens, and prolongs the treatment period. The biologic proporties of antiestrogens can be profoundly altered by their association with some steroid hormones. This is exemplified by

Table 4.11. Relationship between the responses of advanced endometrial adenocarcinoma to successive MPA and tamoxifen treatment. (Adapted from Bonte et al. 1981)

Response to MPA treatment	Response to tamoxifen treatment				
	No. of patients	Complete remission	Partial regression	Stabilization	Progress
Complete regression	4	1	3	0	0
Stabilization	4	0	3	0	1
Unsuccessful adjuvant therapy	4	0	1	0	3

experiments on the chick oviduct, a species in which TAM has very little or no effect on its own (Robel et al. 1986). However, when given together with progesterone and dexamethasone, TAM elicits growth and egg white protein responses similar to those produced by estrogens (Binart et al. 1982; Gravanis et al. 1984). TAM and MPA have been simultaneously added to the culture medium of CG5 cells, a variant of the MCF7 cell line highly sensitive to estrogen (Iacobelli et al. 1983). The inhibition of cell proliferation was higher than that obtained with MPA or TAM alone at a similar dosage. TAM behaves as a pure antiestrogen and the optimal TAM dose maintains PR concentration without, at the same time, significantly increasing tumor growth. In clinical trials using TAM for the treatment of endometrial carcinoma, the dose of TAM should be taken into consideration. Mortel et al. (1985) proposed this view to investigate whether there is a dose at which TAM exhibits different effects on tumor growth and PR levels. Their experimental procedure was as follows: The sex steroid receptor-positive human endometrial carcinoma was transplanted into the nude mice, then groups of animals ($n = 4$) bearing En Ca 101 endometrial carcinoma were subcutaneously implanted with control, estradiol, or TAM pellets: group 1 – control pellets; groups 2–4 – 20 pg/ml, 200 pg/ml, 2 ng/ml estradiol pellets, respectively; groups 5–7 – 2 ng/ml, 20 ng/ml, 200 ng/ml TAM pellets, respectively. Tumor growth was followed up weekly. Tumors were excised and PR concentrations determined. Estradiol showed a dose-dependent increase in the rate of growth of endometrial carcinoma, the greatest increase being observed at 2 ng/ml estradiol concentration. The PR concentrations in tumors exposed to estradiol were about 1200 fmol/mg protein. While TAM increased tumor growth at all doses, the tumor growth rate seen in the presence of a high TAM dose (200 ng/ml) was considerably lower. The PR level in this group, however, remained essentially unchanged (700 fmol/mg protein). Cytosol ER and PR content of the tumor before starting the hormone therapy becomes an essential parameter in conducting the sequential hormonal treatment with TAM and progestogens. The treatment schedule is as follows:

1. ER (+) and PR (+) cancer should first be treated with progestogen administration. This cancer will be transformed to the slightly hormone-responsive ER (+) and PR (−) type after consumption of the cytosol PR reserve. Subsequent TAM administration is needed.
2. ER (+) and PR (−) cancer should first be treated with TAM. TAM can affect the cancer cells by a combined estroantiestrogenic action, depressing the cytosol ER content and inducting PR synthesis, thus overcoming the lack of response to progestogens.
3. ER (−) and PR (−) cancer should also be treated with TAM. In the hormone-independent tumor, TAM seems to act as an estrogen, provoking ER as well as PR synthesis, transforming the caner into hormone-dependent type, and priming this type of cancer for progestogen therapy.

4.4.4 Use of Estrogen After Surgery and Irradiation for Endometrial Carcinoma

One of the historically listed contraindications of hormone replacement is the patient who has received treatment for endometrial carcinoma. In recent years, there have been no data in the literature to suggest the determinable effects of estrogen in these patients. Creasman et al. (1984) reported 163 patients with stage I endometrial adenocarcinoma who were treated at the Duke Medical Center from 1975 to 1980. Thirty patients were given posttreatment estrogen and were compared with 133 patients who did not receive estrogen. Two of thirty (7%) estrogen-treated patients had recurrences compared with 31/133 (23%) of nonestrogen-treated women ($p < 0.05$). It was shown that a history of endometrial carcinoma does not appear to be an absolute contradiction for estrogen replacement therapy.

4.5. Chemotherapy

The use of nonhormonal cytotoxic agents in the treatment of patients with endometrial carcinoma is relatively recent and these nonhormonal cytotoxic agents are mostly employed for recurrent or advanced tumors beyond the control of surgery and radiation and the response to progestogens is expected to be very low. Nonhormonal cytotoxic chemotherapy can offer several advantages; it can control disease in a shorter time than hormonal therapy alone or radiation therapy; it is effective against poorly differentiated cancers which have recurred quickly and are not well treated with other modalities; and it is effective against all sites of recurrence. Nonhormonal cytotoxic agents could be used singly or in combination and both regimes could be used in combination with progestogens.

Routine estrogen receptor (ER) and progesterone receptor (PR) estimation may be helpful in deciding in which patients adjunctive hormone therapy or chemotherapy would be preferable. Recent reports have demonstrated that patients with high concentrations of ER and/or PR respond more frequently to progestin therapy and patients with low concentrations of ER and/or PR have a much lower response to progestin therapy but respond to chemotherapy.

4.5.1 Single-Agent Chemotherapy

The single drugs most frequently studied are 5-fluourouracil (5-FU), cyclophosphamide (CTX), doxorubicin (Adriamycin, ADM), and *cis*-platin (PDD), and the objective response rate varies from 9% to 32% (Deppe 1982).

A series of reports on the objective response rate of single-agent chemotherapy is presented in Table 4.12. It shows that the objective response rate is 19%–38% for ADM, 0%–21% for CTX, and 23% for 5-FU (Thigpen et al. 1979; Devita et al. 1976; Horton et al. 1978). High dose *cis*-platin has an objective response as high as 42% but toxicity forced discontinuation of the treatment in 8 (31%) out of 26 patients (Seski et al. 1982). The single drugs have not been studied adequately and systematically in the past. The optimal dose, administration schedule, and degree of response to the various drugs are unknown.

Christensen et al. (1985) reported the results of determining the optimum conditions in vitro for the use of chemotherapeutic drugs in combination. R1–95 is a cell line obtained from a moderately differentiated endometrial carcinoma which has passed through over 100 generations. It does not respond to progestin. However, the addition of Adriamycin (0.4 $\mu g/ml$) produces 100% inhibition of thymidine uptake (a measure of DNA synthesis) in 24 h and complete cell death within 36 h. The addition of *cis*-platin (2 $\mu g/ml$) produces 83% cell line death and 95% inhibition of thymidine uptake. It is imperative that the optimal therapeutic regimen, including concentration, duration, and sequence of agents, be determined. The knowledge obtained from these in vitro experiments will benefit those patients with endometrial carcinoma receiving combination chemotherapy.

Table 4.12. Single-agent chemotherapy in endometrial carcinoma

			Patients		
			Total	Responding	Response
Series	Year	Drugs	(*n*)	(*n*)	rate (%)
Devita et al.	1976	ADM	18	7	38
		CTX	33	7	21
		5FU	43	10	23
Horton et al.	1978	ADM	21	4	19
		CTX	19	0	0
Thigpen et al.	1979	ADM	43	16	37

4.5.2 Combination Chemotherapy

It seems logical to conclude that combination of effective single agents would improve the response rates in endometrial carcinoma. Bruckner and Deppe (1977) reported that a combination of CTX (500 mg/m^2), ADM (30 mg/m^2), and 5-FU (400 mg/m^2) was administered on the 1st and 8th days every 28 days. MPA (400 mg) was given three times a week intramuscularly. Objective response rate varied from 16% to 37%. CTX, ADM, and PDD (CAP) are a popular combination with a response rate of approximately 57% lasting about 8 months (Deppe 1982). Lovecchio et al. (1984) reported that an overall response rate with 33% complete remission of tumor has been achieved by the combination of CAP-M (CTX, ADM, PDD, MPA). Cohen et al. (1984) reported that 358 patients with advanced FIGO stages III, IV or recurrent endometrial carcinoma were treated with one of two regimens. The objective response rate in those with measurable disease was 36.8% in both groups; 36.8% of each group had stable disease, and only 26.4% progressed with treatment. Response was unaffected by site of recurrence, time of first recurrence, presence or absence of previous treatment with progestational or radiation therapy, or age. Regimen I consisted of melphalan 7 mg/m^2 per day orally for 4 days and 5-FU 525 mg/m^2 per day for 4 days. Both drugs were repeated every 28 days, and 180 mg oral megace was administered daily for 8 weeks and then discontinued.

Regimen II consisted of ADM 40 mg/m^2 i.v. bolus over 5 min, CTX 400 mg/m^2 i.v. bolus over 5 min, and 5-Fu 400 mg/m^2 i.v. bolus over 5 min. All three drugs were repeated every 21 days and 180 mg megace was administered orally daily for 8 weeks and then discontinued.

Ayoub et al. (1986) reported the therapeutic value of adding cyclical hormonal therapy to chemotherapy. A total of 43 patients with advanced endometrial carcinoma were randomized into two groups, regimen A and regimen B. For regimen A, the chemotherapeutic schedule was FAC, i.e., 5-FU 400 mg/m^2 i.v., ADM 30 mg/m^2 i.v., and CTX 400 mg/m^2 i.v., given on the 1st and 8th days every 4 weeks. For regimen B, the schedule was FAC and provera 200 mg daily for 3 weeks followed cyclically by tamoxifen 20 mg daily for 3 weeks. Thirty-six patients were evaluated. In regimen A, 3/15 (20%) had an objective response rate (1 CR + 2 PR) with a median duration of remission of 9.6 months. In regimen B, 9/12 (42.8%) had an objective response rate (5 CR + 4 PR) with a median duration of remission of 20.5 months. A statistical analysis of the results showed a significant difference between the patients treated with chemotherapy only (regimen A) and those receiving chemohormonal therapy (regimen B). Patients with low ER and PR have a higher tendency to relapse which can be significantly diminished by adjuvant cyclical hormonal therapy. A series of reports on combination chemotherapy are presented in Table 4.13. Since the present results of chemotherapy are moderate, it is necessary to study the following areas:

1. Individual selection of dose according to pharmacokinetic parameters.
2. Regional chemotherapy because abdominal or pelvicoabdominal recurrences are frequent and the previous radiotherapy alters tumoral vascularization.

Table 4.13. Combination chemotherapy in endometrial carcinoma

Series	Year	Schedule			Course of treatment
Lloyd et al.	1975	ADM	40 mg/m² i.v.	On the 1st day	
		CTX	200 mg/m² i.v.	On the 3rd–6th days	3 weeks
Bruckner and Deppe	1977	CTX	400 mg/m² i.v.	On the 1st and 8th days	
		ADM	30 mg/m² i.v.	On the 1st and 8th days	
		5FU	400 mg/m² i.v.	On the 1st and 8th days	
		MPA	400 mg i.v.	Twice a week	4 weeks
Muggia et al.	1977	ADM	37.5 mg/m² i.v.	On the 1st day	
		CTX	500 mg/m² i.v.	On the 1st day	3 weeks

3. In vitro or in vivo tests of chemopredictivity.
4. New chemotherapeutic drugs which have stronger effects and fewer side effects could be given.

All these research areas require a multidisciplinary approach to design clinical trials to estimate efficiency, side effects, and indications of chemotherapy. According to this research, chemotherapy will have a better future.

4.6 Suggested Therapy in Each Stage of Endometrial Carcinoma

Surgery alone or in combination with radiation plays a major role in the treatment of the early stage of endometrial carcinoma. Surgical, radiotherapeutic, chemotherapeutic (hormonal or nonhormonal), or a combination of these treatment modalities can be used for treatment of advanced or recurrent disease. For improved survival in endometrial carcinoma individualization is essential in treatment planning. All the different prognostic factors should be available before a final decision is made.

The retrospective study of 418 patients with endometrial carcinoma centered on analyzing the relationship between treatment modalities and prognosis (Li 1988). Based on 30 years of treatment experience in the Cancer Institute Hospital, Beijing and drawing on the latest treatments in other countries in the treatment of endometrial carcinoma, a combined treatment scheme has already been put into effect.

4.6.1 Stage I

Surgery has become routine for the treatment of stage I patients. The proper surgical procedure would be total abdominal hysterectomy, bilateral salpingo-oophorectomy, exploration of pelvic and paraaortic lymph nodes, and selective pelvic and paraaortic lymph node sampling or lymphadenectomy. When one of the following prognostic factors is present, postoperative external radiation may be given. A total dose of 40–45 Gy to the whole pelvis, in general 18×14 cm^2, should be given over 6 weeks.

1. Involvement of the cervical canal
2. Invasion of half or more than one-half of the myometrium
3. Poorly differentiated
4. Adenosquamous carcinoma, clear-cell carcinoma, or papillary adenocarcinoma
5. More extensive tumors outside the uterus

Adjuvant progestogen therapy is necessary provided the peritoneal cytology findings are positive.

4.6.2 Stage II

Patients with stage II endometrial carcinoma may be divided into those with occult (microscopic) or overt (gross) involvement of the cervix. Stage II occult disease should be managed as stage I. In overt stage II disease, preoperative intracavitary irradiation followed by surgery could be considered. A dose of approximately 10–20 Gy intracavitary radiation on point A should be given in two to three fractions, and wide-cuff hysterectomy is performed 7–10 days later. If there are enlarged pelvic lymph nodes or paraaortic lymph nodes, they should be sampled or lymphadenectomy performed. About 40–45 Gy postoperative external whole pelvis irradiation should be given 10–14 days after surgery. If there are paraaortic lymph node metastases, adjuvant external irradiation should be given to this area. In patients with hormone-responsive ER(+) and/or PR(+) carcinoma, progestin administration could be started to last 1 year.

4.6.3 Stages III and IV

If there is the possibility of tumor resection, surgery would seem desirable. Wide-cuff hysterectomy, hysterectomy, and salpingo-oophorectomy or a debulking operation should be performed. If the enlarged uterus was found on pelvic examination, preoperative intracavitary irradiation of 20–30 Gy at point F should be delivered. Pelvic and paraaortic lymph nodes should be sampled. Lymphadenectomy should be considered if it is possible. Postoperative whole pelvis external irradiation of 40–45 Gy should be given. A dose of 40–45 Gy external irradiation to the paraaortic area is used if there are paraaortic lymph node metastases.

If the patients with more extensive tumors are considered technically inoperable, they should be treated with radiotherapy alone. The usual treatment consists of pelvic external irradiation of the parametrium with a midline block to a total of 40–45 Gy and intracavitary irradiation of approximately a total of 40 Gy at point F.

All patients should receive adjuvant hormone therapy or nonhormonal chemotherapy, i.e., progestin administration should be given to last 1 year if stage III patients have hormone-responsive ER(+) and/or PR(+) carcinoma; progestin treatment may last very well if stage IV patients have hormone-responsive ER(+) and/or PR(+) carcinoma. Combination chemotherapy, e.g., CAP (CTX, ADM, PDD) may be given if the patients have hormone-independent ER(−) and/or PR(−) carcinoma.

4.6.4 Recurrent Disease

Recurrence of endometrial carcinoma may be local (50%), distant (28%), or both distant and local (21%), and the recurrence will be detected within 3 years in 76% of patients. The survival of these patients will depend on the site of recurrence and varies from 2% to 12% (Aalders et al. 1984).

4.6.4.1 Treatment for Local Recurrence

The treatment may be surgical, radio-therapeutic, chemotherapeutic (hormonal or non hormonal), or a combination of these modalities. Patients who have been treated with radiation therapy alone and who have recurrent disease in the cervix, uterus, or upper vagina may profit from local extirpation. The vaginal vault recurrences of patients who did not receive radiation previously may be treated with vaginal radiation by a combination of external radiation followed by intravaginal radiation to deliver an additional mucosal dose. Parametrial recurrence in the patients who have previously not received radiation should be treated with whole pelvic radiation. The adjuvant hormone treatment or chemotherapy should be given to each patient who has undergone operation or radiation. All patients who cannot be managed by operation or radiation should receive high-dose progestogen therapy or chemotherapy.

4.6.4.2 Treatment for Distant Metastases

Nearly all patients with distant metastases should receive high-dose progestogen therapy or chemotherapy, i.e., if patients have hormone-responsive ER(+) and/or PR(+) carcinomas, progestin treatment may last very well; if patients have hormone-independent ER(−) and/or PR(−) carcinomas, combination chemotherapy (e.g., CAP) should be administered. If there is no possibility of measuring ER and PR, the hormonal therapy or chemotherapy should be administered depending on the pathogenic characteristic (PC) factors. If the tumor is sensitive to HPC according to the PC factors, prolonged HPC therapy

Table 4.14. Combined treatment planning for patients with primary endometrial carcinoma at the Cancer Institute Hospital, Beijing

Stage of tumor (FIGO)		Preoperative treatment	Operation or irradiation	Adjuvant treatment
I		None	TAH + BSO	Postoperative ExR to pelvis should be given, if patients have one or more high-risk factors. Microscopic cervix involvement; invasion of greater than half the myometrium; grade III adenocarcinoma; adenosquamous carcinoma, clear cell carcinoma; papillary adenocarcinoma; adnexal metastases. 17α-HPC should be used if peritoneal cytology positive
II	Occult	None	TAH + BSO or extended hysterectomy	As stage I
	Overt	Preoperative intracavitary irradiation DT 10–20 Gy at point F	Extended hysterectomy pelvic, paraaortic LN sampling or resection	Whole pelvic ExR, DT 40–45 Gy; paraaortic irradiation, DT 40–45 Gy if paraaortic LN positive; 17α-HPC for 1 year if ER and/or PR positive
III		Intracavitary irradiation, DT 20–30 Gy at point F if uterus enlarged	TAH + BSO or extended or extended hysterectomy or cytoreductive surgery; pelvic, paraaortic LN sampling or resection if surgery indicated; Primary irradiation Pelvic ExR with intracavitary radiation, DT 40 Gy at point F; intravaginal radiation if metastases to vagina	Whole pelvic postoperative ExR, DT 40–45 Gy; Paraaortic irradiation DT 40–45 Gy if paraaortic LN positive; if ER and/or PR positive, HPC therapy for 1 year in stage III, prolonged HPC therapy in stage IV; if ER and PR negative; CAP chemotherapy should be given
IV				

Recurrence	Local	None	TAH+BSO if postradiative uterine recurrence; intracavitary radiation if postoperative or postradiative vaginal recurrence; external pelvic radiation if postoperative parametrial metrial or pelvic recurrence; chemo-or progestogen therapy if surgery and irradiation contraindicated	Postoperative or postradiative chemo- or hormone therapy as stage III–IV
	Distant	None	Prolonged HPC therapy if ER and/or PR positive or the tumor is sensitive to HPC therapy according to PC factors; CAP chemotherapy if ER and PR negative or the tumor is not sensitive to HPC therapy according to PC factors	

TAH + BSO, total hysterectomy and bilateral salpingo-oophrectomy; ExR, external irradiation; 17α-HPC, 17α-hydroxyprogesterone caproate; CAP, CTX, ADM and PDD; DT tissue dose factors, PC pathogenic characteristic factors.

should be given; on the contrary, nonhormonal chemotherapy should be administered.

Combination treatment planning for patients with primary endometrial carcinoma at the Cancer Institute Hospital, Beijing is shown in Table 4.14.

1. The schedule of 17β-hydroxyprogesterone caproate (17β-HPC) therapy in the Cancer Institute Hospital is as follows: 17β-HPC i.m. at a dose of 500 mg/day for 8 weeks, then every 2 days for 8 weeks, then twice a week for 8 weeks, then 500 mg once a week as a maintenance dose.
2. Pathogenic characteristic factors: The premorbid period in such patients is characterized by anovulatory uterine bleeding, infertility, and delayed onset of postmenopausal period. In these patients highly differentiated tumor with superficial invasion into the myometrium develops against the background of hyperplastic endometrium combined with stromal hyperplasia of the ovaries. In these patients metabolic disturbances can be observed: obesity, hyperlipidemia, and decreased tolerance of glucose.

References

Aalders JG, Abeler V, Kolstad P (1984) Recurrent adenocarcinoma of the endometrium: a clinical and histopathological study of 379 patients. Gynecol Oncol 17:85–103

Anderson DG (1965) Management of advanced endometrial adenocarcinoma with medroxyprogesterone acetate. Am J Obstet Gynecol 92:87–97

Anderson DG (1972) The possible mechanisms of action of progestins on endometrial adenocarcinoma. Am J Obstet Gynecol 113:195–211

Annegers J, Malkasian G (1981) Patterns of other neoplasia in patients with endometrial carcinoma. Cancer 48:856–859

Arneson A (1936) Clinical results and histologic changes following the radiation treatment of cancer of the corpus uteri. Am J Roentgenol 36:461

Ayoub J, Audet-Lapointe P, Methot Y et al. (1986) Randomized trial of the addition of cyclical hormonal therapy to combination chemotherapy for advanced endometrial cancer. Gynecol Oncol 23:255

Badib AO, Kurohara SS, Vongtama VY, Webster JH (1969) Evaluation of primary radiation therapy in stage I, group 2 endometrial carcinoma. Radiology 93:417–421

Barni S, Novelli GC, Zanoio L et al. (1981) Chromatin analysis in human endometrial adenocarcinoma before and after treatment with MPA. Virchows Arch (Cell Pathol) 37:167–177

Beck RP, Latour JPA (1963) Necropsy reports on 36 cases of endometrial carcinoma. Am J Obstet Gynecol 85:307–311

Beiler DD, Schmutz DA, O'Rourke TL (1972) Carcinoma of the endometrium: radiation and surgery versus surgery alone. Radiology 102:159–164

Berman ML, Barlow SC, Lagasse LD et al. (1980) Prognosis and treatment of endometrial cancer. Am J Obstet Gynecol 136:679–688

Berman ML, Afridi MA, Kanbour AL, Ball HG (1982) Risk factors and prognosis in stage II endometrial cancer. Gynecol Oncol 14:49–61

Binart N, Mester J, Baulier EE, Catelli MG (1982) Combined effects of progesterone and Tamoxifen in the chick oviduct. Endocrinology 111:7–16

Bojar H, Stusckhe M, Staib W (1983) Effects of high-dose medroxyprogesterone acetate (MPA) on plasma membrane lipid mobility. J Steroid Biochem [Suppl] 19:107

Bokhman JV, Chepick OF, Volkova AT, Vishnevsky AS (1981) Adjuvant hormone therapy of primary endometrial carcinoma with oxyprogesterone caproate. Gynecol Oncol 11:371–378

Bokhman JV, Chepick OF, Volkova AT, Vishnevsky AS (1985) Can primary endometrial carcinoma stage I be cured without surgery and radiation therapy? Gynecol Oncol 20:139–155

Bonte J, Kohorn I (1978) The response of hyperplastic, dysplastic and neoplastic endometrium to progestational therapy. In: Richardson GS, MacLaughlin DT (eds) Hormone biology of endometrial cancer. UICC, Geneva, p 155–184

Bonte J (1979) Developments in endocrine therapy of endometrial and ovarian cancer. Rev Endocrin Relat Cancer 3:11–17

Bonte J (1980) Hormonal dependence of endometrial adenocarcinoma and its hormonal sensitivity to progesterone and antiestrogens. Prog Cancer Res Ther 14:443–455

Bonte J, Ide P, Billiet G, Wynants P (1981) Tamoxifen as a possible chemotherapeutic agent in endometrial adenocarcinoma. Gynecol Oncol 11:140–161

Bonte J (1983) Hormone dependency and hormone responsiveness of endometrial adenocarcinoma to estrogens, progesterone and antiestrogens. In: Campio L, Robustelli G, Cuna D, Taylor RW (eds) Role of medroxyprogesterone in endocrine-related tumors, vol II. Raven, New York, p 141–156

Bonte J (1984) The endometrial adenocarcinoma as a model for hormone-dependency and hormone-responsiveness of gynaecological cancers. Eur J Obstet Gynecol Reprod Biol 18:335–341

Bonte J (1985) Hormone treatment of gynecological tumors. In: Williams CJ, Whitehouse JMA (eds) Cancer investigation and management, vol 3: cancer of the female reproductive system. Wiley, New York, p 141

Boronow RC (1969) Carcinoma of the corpus: treatment at MD Anderson Hospital, in cancer of the uterus and ovary (Anderson Hospital). Year Book Medical Publishers, Chicago, p 35–61

Boronow RC, Morrow CP, Creasman WT et al. (1984) Surgical staging of endometrial cancer: 1. Clinical-pathologic findings of a prospective study. Obstet Gynecol 63:825–838

Broens J, Mouridsen HT, Soerensen HM (1980) Tamoxifen in advanced endometrial carcinoma. Cancer Chemother Pharmacol 4:213

Bruckner HW, Deppe G (1977) Combination chemotherapy of advanced endometrial carcinoma with adriamycin, cyclophosphamide, 5-fluorouracil, and medroxyprogesterone acetate. Obstet Gynecol 50:10–125

Brunschwig A, Murphy AI (1954) The rationale for radical panhysterectomy and pelvic node excision in carcinoma of the corpus uteri. Am J Obstet Gynecol 68:1482–1488

Caffier H, Horner G, Baum RJ (1982) Treatment of advanced or recurrent endometrial adenocarcinoma with progestins, including medroxyprogesterone acetate. In: Proceedings of the international symposium on medroxyprogesterone acetate. Excerpta Medica, Geneva, 389–396

Chau PM (1962) Technic and evaluation of preoperative radium therapy in adenocarcinoma of the uterine corpus. In: Carcinoma of the uterine cervix, endometrium and ovary. Year Book Medical Publishers, Chicago, p 235

Christensen C, Malviya V, Deppe G et al. (1985) RL-95: a model for chemotherapeutic agents in endometrial adenocarcinoma. Gynecol Oncol 20:266

Cohen CJ, Bruckner HW, Deppe G et al. (1984) Multidrug treatment of advanced and recurrent endometrial carcinoma: a gynecologic oncology group study. Obstet Gynecol 63:719–726

Connelly PJ, Alberhasky RC, Christopherson WM (1982) Carcinoma of the endometrium III. Analysis of 865 cases of adenocarcinoma and adenoacanthoma. Obstet Gynecol 59:569–575

Creasman WT, Rutledge FN (1971) The prognostic value of peritoneal cytology in gynecologic malignant disease. Am J Obstet Gynecol 110:773–781

Creasman WT, Weed JC Jr (1981) Carcinoma of endometrium (FIGO Stage I and II): clinical features and management. In: Coppleson M (ed) Gynecologic oncology, fundamental principles and clinical practice. Churchill Livingstone, Edinbourgh, p 571–577

Creasman WT, Boronow RC, Morrow CP et al. (1976) Adenocarcinoma of the endometrium: its metastatic, lymph node potential. Gynecol Oncol 4:239–243

Creasman WT, DiSaia PJ, Blessing T et al. (1981) Prognostic significance of peritoneal cytology in patients with endometrial cancer and preliminary data concerning therapy with intraperitoneal radiopharmaceuticals. Am J Obstet Gynecol 141:921–929

Creasman WT, Henderson D, Clarke-Pearson DL (1984) Use of estrogen after treatment for adenocarcinoma of the endometrium. Gynecol Oncol 17:255

Cullen TH (1900) Cancer of the uterus. Philadelphia, Saunders.

Dahle R (1956) Transtubal spread of tumor cells in carcinoma of the body of the uterus. Surg Gynecol Obstet 102:332

Delclos L, Braun EJ, Herrera JR et al. (1963) Whole abdominal irradiation by cobalt-60 moving-step technic. Radiology 81:632–641

Delclos L, Fletcher GH (1969) Malignant tumors of the endometrium: evaluation of some aspects of radiotherapy, M. D. Anderson Hospital. In: Cancer of the uterus and ovary 11th clinical conference on cancer, M. D. Anderson Hospital and Tumor Institute, Houston, 1966. Year Book Medical Publishers, Chicago, p 62–72

Dembo AJ, Van Dyk J, Japp B et al. (1979) Whole abdominal irradiation by a moving-strip technique for patients with ovarian cancer. Int J Radiat Oncol Biol Phys 5:1933–1942

Deppe G (1982) Chemotherapeutic treatment of endometrial carcinoma. Clin Obstet Gynaecol 25:93–99

Devita VT, Wasserman TH, Young RC, Carter SK (1976) Perspectives on research in gynecologic oncology. Cancer 38:509–525

Dobbie BMW (1953) Vaginal recurrences in carcinoma of the body of the uterus and their prevention by radium therapy. J Obstet Gynecol Br Commonw 60:702–705

Du Toit JP (1985) Carcinoma of the uterine body. In: Shepherd JH, Monaghan JM (eds) Clinical gynecological oncology. Blackwell, Oxford, p 97–132

Enk L, Crona N, Friberg LG et al. (1985) High-dose depot-medroxyprogesterone acetate – effects on the fatty acid composition of serum lecithin and cholesterol ester. Gynecol Oncol 22:317–323

Ferenczy A (1977) Surface ultrastructural response of the human uterine lining epithelium to homonal environment. A scanning electron microscopic study. Acta Cytol 21:566–572

Ferrazzi E, Cartei G, Mattazzo R, Fiorentino M (1977) Oestrogen-like effect of tamoxifen on vaginal epithelium (letter). Br Med J 1:1351–1352

FIGO (1985) Annual report on the results of the treatment in gynecological cancer, vol 18. Statements of results obtained in 1973–1975. Radium hemmet, Stockholm

Frick HC, Munnell EW, Richart RM et al. (1973) Carcinoma of endometrium. Am J Obstet Gynecol 115:663–676

Gagnon JD, Moss WT, Gabourel LS, Stevens KR (1979) External irradiation in the management of stage II endometrial carcinoma. Cancer 44:1247–1251

Geisler HE (1973) The use of megestrol acetate in the treatment of advanced malignant lesions of the endometrium. Gynecol Oncol 1:340

Graham J (1971) The value of preoperative or postoperative treatment by radium for carcinoma of the uterine body. Surg Gynecol Obstet 132:855–860

Gravanis A, Binart P, Robel P et al. (1984) Estrogen-like effects of combined dexamethasone and tamoxifen in the chick oviduct. Biochem Biophys Res Commun 124:57–62

Groom GV, Griffiths K (1976) Effect of the anti-oestrogen tamoxifen on plasma levels of luteinizing hormone, follicle-stimulating hormone, prolactin, oestradiol and progesterone in normal pre-menopausal women. J Endocrinol 70:421–428

Gurpide E, Tseng L (1977) Estrogen metabolism in normal and neoplastic endometrium. Am J Obstet Gynecol 129:809–816

Gurpide E (1979) Hormonal aspects of carcinoma of the endometrium. Gynecol Cancer 8:191–198

Gurpide E (1981) Hormone receptors in endometrial cancer. Cancer 48:638–641

Gusberg SB, Yannopoulos D (1964) Therapeutic decision in corpus cancer. Am J Obstet Gynecol 88:157–162

Hald I (1981) The use of tamoxifen ('Novadex') in endometrial cancer. Rev Endocrin Relat Cancer [Suppl] 8:9–15

Healy WP (1939) Experience with surgical radiation therapy in carcinoma of the corpus uteri. Am J Obstet Gynecol 38:1

Henriksen E (1949) The lymphatic spread of carcinoma of the cervix and of the body of the uterus; a study of 420 necropsies. Am J Obstet Gynecol 58:924–940

Heyman J (1947) Improvement of results in the treatment of uterine cancer. J Am Hosp Ass 135:412–416

Heyman J, Reuterwall O, Beuner S (1941) The Radiumhemmet experience with radiotherapy in cancer of the corpus of the uterus: classification, method of treatment and results. Acta Radiol 22:11–98

Holincka CF, Gurpide E (1980) Peroxidase activity in glands and stroma of human endometrium. Am J Obstet Gynecol 138:599–603

Horton J, Bezz CB, Arsenean J et al. (1978) Comparison of adriamycin with cyclophosphamide in patients with advanced endometrial cancer. Cancer Treat Rep 62:154–161

Iacobelli S, Sica G, Natoli C, Gatti D (1983) Inhibitory effects of medroxyprogesterone acetate on the proliferation of human breast cancer cells. In: Campio L, Robustelli G, Cuna D, Taylor RW (eds) Role of medroxyprogesterone in endocrine-related tumors, vol 2. Raven, New York, p 1–6

Ishiwata I, Nozawa S, Okumura H (1977) Effects of 17β-estradiol and progesterone on growth and morphology of human endometrial carcinoma cells in vitro. Cancer Res 37:4246–4249

Janne O (1979) Female sex steroid receptors in normal hyperplastic and carcinomatous endometrium. The relationship to serum steroid hormones and gonadotropins and changes during medroxyprogesterone acetate administration. Int J Cancer 24:545–554

Jones HW (1975) Treatment of adenocarcinoma of the endometrium. Obstet Gynecol Surv 30:147–169

Jordan VC, Dix CJ (1978) Effect of estradiol benzoate, tamoxifen and monohydroxy-tamoxifen on immature rat uterine progesterone receptor synthesis and endometrial cell division. J Steroid Biochem 11:285–291

Joslin CAF (1985) The place for radiotherapy in endometrial cancer. Proceedings of International Meeting of Gynaecological Oncology, Venice-Lido (Italy) Apr 1985, p 21–24

Joslin CAF, Vaishampayan GV, Mallik T (1977) The treatment of early cancer of the corpus uteri. Radiology 50:38–45

Kadar NRD, Kohorn EI, LiVolsi VA, Kapp DS (1982) Histologic variants of cervical involvement by endometrial carcinoma. Obstet Gynecol 59:85–92

Kauppila A, Fribert LG (1981) Hormone and cytotoxic chemotherapy for endometrial carcinoma. Acta Obstet Gynecol Scand [Suppl] 101:59–64

Kauppila A, Gronroos M, Niemineu U (1982) Clinical outcome of endometrial cancer. Obstet Gynecol 60:473–480

Keettel WC, Pixley EE, Buchsbaum HJ (1974) Experience with peritoneal cytology in the management of gynecological malignancies. Am J Obstet Gynecol 120:174–182

Kelley RM (1951) Proceedings of the second conference on steroids and cancer, Council on Pharmacy and Chemistry, American Medical Association Chicago, 116

Kelley RM, Baker WH (1961) Progestational agents in the treatment of carcinoma of the endometrium. N Engl J Med 264:216–222

Kennedy A Peterson G, Becker S, Webster K (1986) Experience with pelvic washings in stage I and II endometrial adenocarcinoma. Gynecol Oncol 23:256

Kinsella TJ, Bloomer WD, Lavin PT et al. (1980) Stage II endometrial carcinoma: ten year follow up combined radiation and surgical treatment. Gynecol Oncol 11:290–297

Kistner RW, Griffiths CT, Craig JM (1965) Use of progestational agents in the management of endometrial cancer. Cancer 18:1563–1579

Kjellgren O, Magnusson SS (1970) Efficacy of primary radiation in carcinoma of the endometrium. Acta Radiol 9:102–104

Kohorn EI (1976) Gestagens and endometrial carcinoma. Gynecol Oncol 4:398–411

Lampe I (1963) Endometrial carcinoma. Am J Roentgenol 90:1011–1015

Laatikainen T, Nieminea U, Adlercreutz H (1979) Plasma medroxyprogesterone acetate levels following intramuscular or oral administration in patients with endometrial adenocarcinoma. Acta Obstet Gynecol Scand 58:85–99

Lewis B, Stallworthy JA, Cowdell R (1970) Adenocarcinoma of the body of the uterus. J Obstet Gynecol Br Commonw 77:343–348

Lewis GC, Slack NH et al. (1974) Adjuvant progestogen therapy in the primary definitive treatment of endometrial cancer. Gynecol Oncol 2:368–376

Li SY (1988) Treatment. In: Li SY (ed) Endometrial carcinoma. People's Medical Publishing House, Beijing, p 94–168

Lloyd RE, Jones SE, Sammon SE (1975) Southwest oncology group members: "Phase II trial of adriamycin and cyclophosphamide: a southwest oncology group pilot study". Proc Am Assoc Cancer Res 16:265

Lovecchio JL, Averette HE, Lichtinger M et al. (1984) Treatment of advanced or recurrent endometrial adenocarcinoma with cyclophosphamide, doxorubicin, cis-platinum and megestrol acetate. Obstet Gynecol 63:557–560

Malkasian GD, Decker DG, Mussey E, Johnson CG (1971) Progestin treatment of recurrent endometrial carcinoma. Am J Obstet Gynecol 110:15–23

Marchesoni D, Mozzanega B, Gangemi M, Enrichi H (1980) Tamoxifen in the therapy of post-menopausal endometrial cancer: variations in some hormonal parameters. Eur J Gynaecol Oncol 1:116–121

Marcial VA, Tome JM, Ubinas J (1969) The combination of external irradiation and curietherapy used preoperatively in adenocarcinoma of the endometrium. Am J Roentgenol Nucl Med 105:586–595

Martin PM, Rolland PH, Jacquemier J et al. (1979) Multiple steroid receptors in human breast cancer. II. Estrogen and progesterone receptors in 672 primary tumors. III. Relationship between steroid receptors and the state of differentiation and the activity of carcinomas throughout the pathologic feature. Cancer Chemother Pharmacol 2:107–120

Masson JC, Gregg RD (1940) Carcinoma of the body of the uterus: experience of the Mayo Clinic for 24 years. Surg Gynecol Obstet 70:1083

McCabe JG, Sagerman RH (1979) Treatment of endometrial cancer in a regional radiation therapy center. Cancer 43:1052–1057

McGrew EA, Laws JF, Coles WH (1954) Free malignant cells in relation to recurrence of carcinoma of the colon. JAMA 154:1251

Milton PJD, Metters JS (1972) Endometrial carcinoma – an analysis of 355 patients treated at St. Thomas' Hospital, 1945-1969. J Obstet Gynecol Br Commonw 79:455–464

Moazzami B, Van der Walt JD, Boyd NR (1983) Use of progestogens as an adjuvant to surgery in the treatment of stage I adenocarcinoma of the uterine corpus. Br J Obstet Gynaecol 90:178–181

Morrow CP, DiSaia PJ, Townsend DE (1973) Current management of endometrial carcinoma. Obstet Gynecol 42:399–406

Morrow CP, Townsend DE (1981) Cancer of the uterine corpus. In: Synopsis of gynecologic oncology. Wiley, New York, p 133

Morrow CP, Schlaerth JB (1982) Surgical management of endometrial carcinoma. Clin Obstet Gynecol 25:81–92

Morrow CP, Creasman WT, Homesley H et al. (1986) Recurrence in endometrial carcinoma as a function of extended surgical staging data (a gynecological oncology group study). In: Morrow CP, Smart Ge (eds) Gynecological oncology. Springer Berlin Heidelberg New York, p 147–153

Mortel R, Levy C, Welff JP et al. (1981) Female sex steroid receptors in postmenopausal endometrial carcinoma and biochemical response to an antiestrogen. Cancer 41:1140–1147

Mortel R, Zaino R, Satyaswaroop PG (1984) Response of endometrial carcinoma to sequential treatment with tamoxifen and progestin in the Nude Mouse Model. Gynecol Oncol 17:253–254

Mortel R, Zaino RJ, Satyaswaroop PG (1985) Response of human endometrial carcinoma to various doses of estradiol and tamoxifen in the nude mouse model. Gynecol Oncol 20:257

Muggia FM, Chia GA, Reed LJ, Romney SL (1977) Doxorubicin-cyclophosphamide: effective therapy for advanced endometrial cancer. Am J Obstet Gynecol 128:314–319

Nahhas WA, Whitney CW, Stryker JA et al. (1980) Stage II endometrial carcinoma. Gynecol Oncol 10:303–311

Nahhas WA, Zaino R, Mortel R (1984) Residual carcinoma in the surgical specimen of patients with endometrial adenocarcinoma undergoing preoperative radiation therapy. A study of 80 patients and a literature review. Gynecol Oncol 18:165–176

Onsrud M, Kolstad P, Normann T (1976) Postoperative external pelvic irradiation in carcinoma of the corpus stage I: a controlled clinical trial. Gynecol Oncol 4:222–231

Pannutti F (1981) High doses of medroxyprogesterone acetate in advanced cancer treatment. Plasma levels and bioavailability after single and multiple dose administration, preliminary results. In symposium: role of medroxyprogesterone acetate in endocrine-related tumors, 1981 Rome.

Park R, Patow W, Petty W, Zimmermann E (1974) Treatment of adenocarcinoma of the endometrium. Gynecol Oncol 2:60–70

Paterson R (1948) The treatment of malignant disease by radium and X-rays: being a practice of radiotherapy. Arnold, London p 249–432

Piver MS, Yazigi R, Blumenson LE, Tsukada Y (1979) A prospective trial comparing hysterectomy, hysterectomy plus vaginal radium, and uterine radium plus hysterectomy in stage I endometrial carcinoma. Obstet Gynecol 54:85–89

Piver MS (1980) Stage I endometrial carcinoma: the role of adjunctive radiation therapy. Int J Radiat Oncol Biol Phys 6:367–368

Piver MS, Barlow JJ, Lurain JR, Blumenson LE (1980) Medroxyprogesterone acetate (Depo-provera) Vs hydroxyprogesterone caproate (Delalutin) in women with metastatic endometrial adenocarcinoma. Cancer 45:268–272

Piver MS, Lele SB, Barlow JJ et al. (1982) Para-aortic lymph node evaluation in stage I endometrial carcinoma. Obstet Gynecol 59:97–100

Prodi G, Nicoletti G, DeGiovanni C et al. (1980) Multiple steroid hormone receptors in normal and abnormal human endometrium. J Cancer Res Clin Oncol 98:173–183

Quinn MA, Campbell JJ, Murray R, Pepperell RJ (1981) Tamoxi fen and aminoglute-thimide in the management of patients with advanced endometrial carcinoma not responsive to medroxyprogesterone. Aust NZ J Obstet Gynaecol 21:226–227

Randall JH, Goddard WBA (1956) A study of 531 cases of endometrial carcinoma. Surg Gynecol Obstet 103:221–226

Reel JR (1976) The mode of action of progestagens on endometrial carcinoma. In: Steroid hormone action and cancer, vol 4, W 1 CU 82M. Plenum, New York, p 85–94

Reifenstein EC (1974) The treatment of advanced endometrial cancer with hydroxy-progesterone caproate. Gynecol Oncol 2:377–414

Ritcher N, Lucas WE, Yon JL, Sanford GD (1981) Preoperative whole pelvic external irradiation in stage I endometrial cancer. Cancer 48:58–62

Robel P, Levy C, Bayard F et al. (1979) Estradiol and progesterone receptors in normal and abnormal human endometrium. In: Klopper et al. (eds) Research on steroids, vol VIII. Academic, London, p 77–85

Robel P, Gravanis A, Roger-Jallais L et al. (1986) Receptors, hormones and anti-hormones in postmenopausal endometrial carcinoma. In: Bolla M, Racinet C, Vrousos C (eds) Endometrial cancers. 5th Cancer Research Workshop, Grenoble 1985. Karger, Basel, p 119–125

Rutledge FN (1974) The role of radical hysterectomy in adenocarcinoma of the endometrium. Gynecol Oncol 2:331–347

Rutledge FN, Tan SK, Fletcher GM (1958) Vaginal metastasis from adenocarcinoma of the corpus uteri. Am J Obstet Gynecol 75:167–174

Sala JM, Del Regato JA (1961) Treatment of carcinoma of the endometrium. Radiology 79:12–17

Salazar OM, Feldstein ML, DePapp EW et al. (1978) The management of clinical stage I endometrial carcinoma. Cancer 41:1016–1026

Salimtschik M, Mouridsen HT, Loeber J, Johansson E (1980) Comparative pharma-cokinetics of MPA administered by oral and i.m. route. Cancer Chemother Pharmacol 4:267–269

Sall S, Sonnenblick B, Stone ML (1970) Factors affecting survival of patients with endometrial adenocarcinoma. Am J Obstet Gynecol 107:116–123

Sall S, DiSaia P, Morrow CP et al. (1979) A comparison of medroxyprogesterone serum concentrations by the oral or intramuscular route in patients with persistent or recurrent endometrial carcinoma. Am J Obstet Gynecol 135:647–650

Satyaswaroop PG, Frost A, Gurpide E (1980) Metabolism and effects of progesterone in the human endometrial adenocarcinoma cell line HEC-1. Steroids 35:21–37

Seski JC, Edwards CL, Herson J et al. (1982) Cisplatin chemotherapy in disseminated endometrial cancer. Obstet Gynecol 59:225–228

Shimm DS, Wang CC, Fuller AF et al. (1986) Management of high-grade stage I adenocarcinoma of the endometrium: hysterectomy following low dose external beam pelvic irradiation. Gynecol Oncol 23:183–191

Silverberg SG, DeGiorgi LS (1974) Histopathologic analysis of preoperative radiation therapy in endometrial carcinoma. Am J Obstet Gynecol 119:698–704

Smith JP, Rutledge F, Soffar SW (1966) Progestins in the treatment of patients with endometrial adenocarcinoma. Am J Obstet Gynecol 94:977–984

Strickland P (1965) Carcinoma corporis uteri: a radical intracavitary treatment. Clin Radiol 16:112–118

Suit HD, Shalek RJ (1963) Response of anoxic C3H mouse mammary carcinoma isotransplants (1–25 mm³) to X irradiation. JNCI 31:479–495

Suit HD, Gallager HS (1964) Intact tumor cells in irradiated tissue. Arch Pathol 78:648–651

Surwit EA, Joelsson I, Einhorn N (1981) Adjunctive radiation therapy in the management of stage I cancer of the endometrium. Obstet Gynecol 58:590–595

Sutherland RL, Mester J, Baulieu EE (1977) Tamoxifen is a potent pure antiestrogen in chick oviduct. Nature 267:434–435

Swenerton KD, Shaw D, White GW, Boyes DA (1979) Treatment of advanced endo-metrial carcinoma with tamoxifen. N Engl J Med 301:105

Swenerton KD (1980) Treatment of advanced endometrial adenocarcinoma with tamoxi-fen. Cancer Treat Rep 64:805–811

Tamassia V, Battaglia A, Ganzina F et al. (1982) Pharmacokinetic approach to selection of dose schedules for MPA in clinical oncology. Cancer Chemother Pharmacol 8:151–156

Tamassia V (1986) Clinical pharmacokinetics of medroxyprogesterone acetate: relevance for the treatment of breast and endometrial cancer. In: Bolla M, Racinet C, Vrousos C (eds) Endometrial cancers. 5th Cancer Research Workshop, Grenoble 1985. Karger, Basel, p 168–176

Taylor HC Jr, Becker WF (1947) Carcinoma of the corpus uteri: end-results of treatment in 531 cases from 1926–1940. Surg Gynecol Obstet 84:129–139

Thigpen JT, Buchsbaum HJ, Mangan C, Blessing JA (1979) Phase II trial of adriamycin in the treatment of advanced or recurrent endometrial carcinoma: a gynecologic oncology group study. Cancer Treat Rep 63:21–27

Thigpen JT, Blessing JA, DiSaia P, Ehrlich C (1985) Treatment of advanced or recurrent endometrial carcinoma with medroxyprogesterone acetate (MPA): a gynecologic oncology group study. Gynecol Oncol 20:250

Truskett ID, Constable WC (1968) Management of carcinoma of the corpus uteri. Am J Obstet Gynecol 101:689–694

Tseng L, Gusberg S, Gurpide E (1977) Estradiol receptor and 17-beta-dehydrogenase in normal and abnormal human endometrium. Ann NY Acad Sci 286:190–198

Varga A, Henriksen E. (1965) Histologic observations on the effect of 17-alpha-hydroxyprogesterone-17-N-caproate on endometrial carcinoma. Obstet Gynecol 26:656–664

Vesterinen E, Backas NE, Pesonen K et al. (1981) Effect of medroxyprogesterone acetate on serum levels of LH, FSH, cortisol and estrone in patients with endometrial carcinoma. Arch Gynecol 230:205–211

Vihko R, Jänne O, Kauppila A (1980) Steroid receptors in normal hyperplastic and malignant human endometria. Ann Clin Res 12:208–215

Vongtama V, Kurohara SS, Badib AO, Webster JH (1970) Second primary cancer of endometrial carcinoma. Cancer 26:842–846

Wait RB (1973) Megestrol acetate in the management of advanced endometrial carcinoma. Obstet Gynecol 41:129–136

Wentz WB (1964) Effect of a progestational agent on endometrial hyperplasia and endometrial cancer. Obstet Gynecol 24:370–375

Wentz WB (1974) Progestin therapy in endometrial hyperplasia. Gynecol Oncol 2:362–367

Wharam MD, Phillips TL, Bagshaw MA (1976) Role of radiation therapy in clinical stage I carcinoma of the endometrium. Int J Radiat Oncol Biol Phys 1:1081–1089

Wintz H (1941) Ergebnisse der Behandlug von Unterleibkrebsen mit Rontgenstrahlen, Strahlentherapie 69:3

Yasizi R, Piver MS, Blumenson L (1983) Malignant peritoneal cytology as prognostic indicator in stage I endometrial cancer. Obstet Gynecol 62:359–362

5 Prognosis of Endometrial Carcinoma

5.1 Treatment Result

In the FIGO Annual Report (1985), 5-year survival was 67.7% in 13 581 cases of endo-metrial carcinoma (Table 5.1). The reported figures of survival have been consistent, ranging from 66% to 77% (Frick et al. 1973; Morrow et al. 1973; Berman et al. 1980; Connelly et al. 1982; Kauppila et al. 1982). Li (1988), reviewing 418 cases of endometrial carcinoma, found 5-year survival to be 77.6% for stage I, 59.6% for stage II, and 61.9% for stages I–IV respectively. The low mortality is probably related to the fact that over 80% of the cases were confined to the uterus (FIGO stages I, II) at initial diagnosis and approximately 75% of cases could be treated by surgery and/or radiotherapy.

5.2 Recurrence

The definition of recurrence is defined as regrowth of the endometrial carcinoma after an apparently complete remission following primary treatment and lasting at least 3 months. Patients with residual disease after the initial treatment are recognized as uncontrolled.

5.2.1 Recurrence Rate

The incidence of recurrence may be 10%–20% in patients with endometrial carcinoma (Nahhas et al. 1971; Milton and Metters 1972; Boutselis 1978; Gusberg 1978). Wu et al. (1982) in the Union Hospital of Beijing have observed that the recurrence rate was 14.5% from 76 followed-up patients. Another report from China showed a recurrence rate of 17.9% (75/418 cases) (Li SY 1988). Failure of adequate local treatment or presence of undetectable tumor cells outside the primary field of treatment may be possible origins of recurrent endometrial carcinoma (Aalders et al. 1984a).

5.2.2 Interval Between Primary Treatment and Recurrence

Within 3 years after completion of the primary treatment, 88.3% of recurrences appeared in 77 patients with endometrial carcinoma (Milton and Metters 1972). Recurrence was detected within 3 years in 81.8% and 90.5% of patients in two

Table 5.1. Endometrial carcinoma: 1976–1978 5-year result. (Adapted from FIGO 1985, p. 128)

	Patients	
	(*n*)	(%)
Five-year survival	**9,192**	67.7
Died of carcinoma of the corpus	**3,048**	22.4
Lost to follow-up	514	3.8
Died from intercurrent disease	827	6.1
Total	**13,581**	100.0

groups, one in the Union Hospital and Cancer Institute Hospital, Beijing (Wu et al 1982; Li 1988). Obviously the majority of recurrences could be detected within 3 years. The recurrence rate will decrease rapidly if recurrence is not detected 5 years after completion of the primary treatment.

5.2.3 Recurrence Location

Recurrence of endometrial carcinoma may be local, distant, or both distant and local. Local recurrence is defined as tumor regrowth anywhere in the pelvic structures or in the lymph nodes located below the pelvic brim. Distant metastases were diagnosed on objective evidence such as palpation of hard enlarged tumor (upper abdomen), nodular enlargement of the liver and lymph nodes (supraclavicular), radiographic signs of progressive solitary or multiple lung metastases, mediastinal or hilar node enlargement, bone destruction, and presence of ascites with malignant cells. The diagnosis is based on clinical and/or radiologic evidence and histologic or cytologic examination (Aalders et al. 1984a). Vaginal involvement may be found in 8.2%–14.7% of patients (Plentl and Friedman 1971; Boutselis 1978; Gusberg 1978). Involvement of the lower vagina is usually due to hematogenous spread while vault recurrence probably represents local extension of implantation at the time of operation. In recent years, with the wider employment of radiation therapy as an adjuvant to hysterectomy, the incidence of isolated vaginal recurrence has diminished significantly. In the Norwegian Radium Hospital, Norway, local recurrence was found in 50% of the patients (190/379 cases), distant metastases in 28% of the patients with recurrences (108/379 cases), and simultaneous local recurrence and distant metastases in 21% of the patients with recurrences (81/379 cases) (Aalders et al. 1984a). In a study of 75 patients with recurrent endometrial carcinoma in the Cancer Institute Hospital, of Beijing, local recurrence was found in 37 patients (nearly 50%) and local recurrence and distant metastases were found in only 6 (8%) (Li SY 1988).

5.2.4 Treatment and Prognosis of Recurrence

The treatment of recurrent disease can be surgical, radiotherapeutic, chemotherapeutic (hormonal or nonhormonal), or a combination of these treatment modalities. The patient with recurrent endometrial carcinoma will respond best to individualized treatment plans. Radiation therapy may be used for the treatment of 64% of recurrent diseases, and surgery may be used for the treatment of only 6%. The prognosis will be better if the recurrent tumor is resected completely.

Aalders et al. (1984a) reported that all untreated patients died in 36 months, but 31% of the treated patients were still alive and at 5 years their survival rate was 13%. Li et al. (1988) at the Cancer Institute Hospital, Beijing observed that 15 of the 30 untreated patients (50%) and 38 of the 45 treated patients (84.4%) were alive at the end of 6 months, but only 1 of the 30 untreated patients (3.4%) was still alive at 5 years. The 5-year survival rate was 24.4% for the treated patients. It is obvious that there is a significant difference between the treated and untreated patients in their prognoses of recurrent endometrial carcinoma. Therefore, careful treatment should be given to recurrent diseases. The prognosis of recurrent endometrial carcinoma is usually very poor. Part of the reason must be attributable to inadequate treatment because radiotherapy in many cases could not be used as it had already been part of the primary treatment. Therefore the optimal primary treatment of endometrial carcinoma has to be decided carefully and thoroughly.

5.3 Prognostic Factors

On the basis of clinical experience, Nolan and Huen (1976) developed a mathematical formula for the evaluation of prognosis which is directly proportional to host resistance factors and inversely proportional to tumor virulence factors.

$$\text{Prognosis } \frac{\alpha = \text{signal of the direct ratio resistance}}{\text{virulence}} \times \text{treatment}$$

The resistance factors are age and general constitutional condition. The virulence factors are stage, grade of tumor, and tumor volume. The prognosis will be directly related to age, general constitutional condition of the patient, stage of disease, grade of tumor, tumor volume, and treatment factors.

5.3.1 Age

Endometrial carcinoma is primarily a disease of postmenopausal women. Only 20%–25% of endometrial carcinomas occur in premenopausal women (Mattingly 1977; Malkasian et al. 1980). The significance of age at the time of diagnosis has been recognized. Frick et al. (1973) found that the survival rate of a group of 261 cases of stage I disease patients under the age of 59 years was better than in a group of older patients. The survival rate was more than 80% for patients below 59 years of age and less than 56% for patients over 60 years of age. Li et al. (1988) reported that the 5-year survival was 89.4% for women below 50 years of age and 54.7% for women over aged 50 years. Wu et al. (1982) noted similar results in their review.

The younger the patient, the better the prognosis, and the older the patient, the worse the prognosis. The improved survival in younger patients is related to the tendency toward earlier, better differentiated lesions with no or very superficial myometrial invasion (Jones 1975; Silverberg and Makowski 1975; Ostor et al. 1982). In older patients, adenocarcinoma grade III, adenosquamous carcinoma, or clear cell carcinoma tend to occur and may influence the prognosis (Aalders et al. 1980) (Tables 5.2, 5.3).

5.3.2 Clinical Stages

According to the FIGO Annual Report (1985), the vast majority of patients complained of stage I disease, with an overall survival of 67.7% (Table 5.4). The

Table 5.2. Grade of differentiation in 10 234 cases of adenocarcinoma of endometrial carcinoma. Mean age by stage and grade of differentiation 1976–1978. (Adapted from FIGO 1985, p. 127)

Grade of differentiation	Stage I	Stage II	Stage III	Stage IV	No stage
Grade I	60.6	61.9	62.8	66.5	67.0
Grade 2	63.1	64.3	64.5	65.3	67.4
Grade 3	64.1	65.7	64.6	65.8	64.9
Not graded	63.3	63.6	64.8	66.2	68.3

Table 5.3. Grade of differentiation in 473 cases of adenosquamous and clear cell carcinoma of the endometrium. Mean age by stage and grade of differentiation (1976–1978). (Adapted from FIGO 1985, p. 127)

Grade of differentiation	Stage I	Stage II	Stage III	Stage IV	No stage
Grade 1	59.8	62.4	57.3	50.5	–
Grade 2	61.2	65.5	65.3	64.8	–
Grade 3	63.2	60.8	66.7	64.9	–
Not graded	62.1	64.9	67.1	63.5	–

Table 5.4. Endometrial carcinoma: FIGO staging versus 5-year survival

	Stage									
	I		II		III		IV		Overall	
Series	(n)	(%)	(n)	(%)	(n)	(%)	(n)	(%)	(n)	(%)
Frick et al. 1973	261	76	22	36	34	44	31	3	248	66.1
Morrow et al. 1973	1860	76	20.5	51	245	26	113	9	2423	68.0
Berman et al. 1980	9670	76	1089	50	480	30	54	9	11293	66.3
Kauppila et al. 1982	845	78	187	61	62	29	19	5	1113	71.0
Connelly et al. 1982	(–)	81	(–)	41	(–)	42	(–)	9	(–)	77.1
Li 1988	228	77.6	105	59.6	76	27.3	9	0	418	61.9

Table 5.5. Endometrial carcinoma, 1976–1978. Distribution by stage and 5-year survival in different stages. (Adapted from FIGO 1985, p. 128)

	Patients treated		Five-year survival	
Stage	(n)	(%)	(n)	(%)
I	10 285	75.7	7729	75.1
II	1 885	13.9	1089	57.8
III	844	6.2	253	30.0
IV	452	3.3	48	10.6
No. stage	115	0.9	73	63.5
Total	13 581	100.0	9192	67.7

5-year survival in patients with different stages was 76%–81% in patients with state I, 36%–61% in patients with stage II, and 26%–44% and 0%–9% in patients with stage III and stage IV respectively (Frick et al. 1973; Morrow et al. 1973; Berman et al. 1980; Connelly et al. 1982; Kauppila et al. 1982; Li et al. 1988) (Table 5.5). It is well known that the more the tumor advances the poorer the prognosis. Unfortunately, it is a disease not readily detectable with cervicovaginal pap smear and none of the present routine cytologic methods have a diagnostic accuracy that approaches that of cytologic screening in cervical cancer.

5.3.3 Lymph Node Involvement

Lymph node involvement has been considered an important factor of tumor virulence. The local invasion of tumor such as myometrial invasion provides the carcinoma with access to the lymphatic channel leading to lymphatic spread and then to hematogenous spread (Yoonessi et al. 1979). Since abdominal total hysterectomy and bilateral salpingo-oophorectomy have been selected as the major methods of treatment and radical hysterectomy or pelvic lymphadenectomy can only be used in some patients, the ture incidence of lymph node involvement has been difficult to determine.

Reviews in the literature reported pelvic node involvement varying from 5.4% to 11.2% in stage I endometrial carcinoma (Morrow et al. 1973; Creasman et al. 1976). In stage II disease, the incidence of lymph node involvement varies from 18.7% to 40% (Hawksworth 1964; Morrow et al. 1973).

Rutledge (1974) in his review of the role of radical hysterectomy in endometrial carcinoma during the period 1950–1973 noted that approximately 10% of patients with stage I carcinoma had metastases to the pelvic nodes. Some of the studies reported a higher incidence of lymphatic node metastases but this was explained by the selection of patients (Table 5.6). Creasman et al. (1976) reported the results of a study by the Gynecologic Oncology Group (GOG) in America, in which 11.4% and 5.7% of a group of 206 patients with stage I disease had one or more pelvic lymph nodes and paraaortic lymph nodes involved.

More recently, paraaortic lymph nodal metastases have been accepted as the most important prognostic factor. Manetta et al. (1986) reported the correlation between paraaortic lymph node involvement and the histologic grade of the tumor and the depth of myometrial invasion in a study of 36 patients with stage I disease. Paraaortic lymph node metastases were directly related to differentiation of the tumor and depth of myometrial invasion (Table 5.7). Morrow et al. in 1986 presented their data concerning stage I endometrial carcinoma and the incidence of lymph node metastases. It is noted that 1% of patients had pelvic node metastases if there was histologic grade I but no myometrial invasion; 40% of the patients had pelvic node metastases if there was histologic grade III and myometrial invasion in the outer third (Table 5.8). Ng and Reagan (1970) presented the correlation between the 5-year survival and differentiation of the tumor and depth of myometrial invasion. The 5-year survival was 90% in patients with grade I but without myometrial invasion, it was only 14% in patients with grade IV and deep myometrial invasion and no one survived in patients with grade III or grade IV and myometrial invasion to the surface of the uterus (Table 5.9).

The incidence of lymph node metastases increased when the tumor was more undifferentiated and penetrated further into the myometrium, and the 5-year survival showed an obvious decrease.

5.3.4 Myometrial Invasion

The depth of myometrial invasion is associated with the other poor prognostic factors, poor differentiation, and lymph node involvement (Table 5.10) (Creasman et al. 1976; Berman 1980; DiSaia and Creasman 1981; Baram et al. 1985).

Table 5.6. Endometrial carcinoma: frequency of lymph node metastases. (Adapted from Rutledge 1974)

Author	Year	Patients with positive nodes (n)	(%)	Stage I	Stage II
Randall	1950	4/20	20%	Not stated	Not stated
Brunschwig	1954	10/57	17%		
Liu and Meigs	1955	11/47	23%	4/33 (12%)	7/14 (50%)
Lefevre	1956	7/45	16%	Not stated	Not stated
Schwartz and Brunschwig	1957	13/96	14%		
Roberts	1961	10/34	29%	5/22 (23%)	2/8 (25%)
Anderson and Stephens	1961	4/52	8%	Not stated	Not stated
Barber et al.	1962	12/85	20%		
Davis	1964	7/56	12.5%	Not stated	Not stated
Parsons	1959	4/50	8%		
Hawksworth	1964	8/64	12.5%		6/11 (18.7%)
Winterton	1964	8/76	10%		
Rickford	1968	5/50	10%	2/36	2/9
Lees	1969	13/76	17%	3/56	4/8
Morris	1967	4/21	20%	16	5
Lewis	1970	17/129	13.2%	12/107 (11.2%)	5/22 (23%)
Stallworthy	1973	18/131	14%		11/27 (40%)

Table 5.7. Stage I endometrial carcinoma. Histologic grade and myometrial invasion versus paraaortic lymph node involvement. (Adapted from Manetta et al. 1986)

Grade and myometrial invasion	Patients (n)	Patients with positive nodes	
		(n)	(%)
G_1	17	1	5.8
G_2	11	0	0
G_3	8	4	50
Inner third	22	1	4.5
Middle third	3	1	33.0
Outer third	7	3	42.8

Table 5.8. Stage I endometrial carcinoma. Histologic grade and myometrial invasion versus pelvic lymph node involvement. (Adapted from Morrow et al. 1986, p. 149)

Histologic grade	Muscle invasion							
	None		Inner third		Middle third		Outer third	
	(n)	(%)	(n)	(%)	(n)	(%)	(n)	(%)
1	1/77	1	2/85	2	1/20	5	3/15	20
2	1/19	5	5/91	5	7/15	14	11/53	21
3	0/11	–	4/35	11	3/18	7	21/53	40

Table 5.9. Stage I endometrial carcinoma. Histologic grade and myometrial invasion versus 5-year survival. (Adapted from Ng and Reagan 1970)

Myometrial invasion	Patients (n)	Broders' grade			
		1 (%)	2 (%)	3 (%)	4 (%)
Endometrium only	129	95	93	64	63
<half	48	92	73	50	50
>half	22	33	38	25	14
Extrauterine involvement	14	33	20	0	0

Table 5.10. Stage I endometrial carcinoma. Myometrial invasion versus pelvic lymph node involvement

Series	Myometrial invasion		
	< third	Middle third	Outer third
Creasman et al. (1976)	7.5%	10.0%	43.0%
Berman et al. (1980)	3.0%	14.0%	41.0%
DiSaia and Creasman (1981)	5.5%	13.3%	46.4%

A review of 15 individual studies in the literature demonstrated a decrease in survival rates from 95% to 34% as myometrial invasion increased (Corscaden and Tovell 1954; Gusberg and Yannopoulos 1964; Climie and Rachmaninoff 1965; Austin and MacMahon 1969; Cheon 1969; Nilson and Koller 1969; Vongtama et al. 1970; Lewis et al. 1970; Sall et al. 1970; Welander et al. 1972; Frick 1973; Keller et al. 1974; Homesley et al. 1976; Li 1988) (Table 5.11). The deeper the myometrial invasion, the lower the eventual survival.

It has been difficult to assess myometrial invasion accurately in the following conditions:

1. In patients who received preoperative irradiation, the assessment of the degree of myometrial invasion is more difficult or is sometimes impossible (Aalders et al. 1980; Surwit et al. 1981).
2. The problem of the coexistence of endometrial carcinoma and adenomyosis has been addressed by several authors. The incidence of adenomyosis in endometrial carcinoma ranges from 1.4% to 60% (Giammalvo and Kaplan 1958; Emge 1962; Marcus 1962; Weed et al. 1966; Molitor 1971; Greenwood 1976; Owelabi and Strickler 1977; Hernandez and Woodruff 1980). In most cases, assessment of the extent of myometrial invasion is not a difficult problem. However, when the carcinoma involves the foci of adenomyosis extensively, the distinction between adenomyosis and myometrial invasion of tumor may be difficult. The prognosis of the tumor involving adenomyosis is different from that of myometrial invasion of the tumor. Hall et al. (1984) reported that the 5-year survival was 96% (50/52 cases) in patients with stage I endometrial carcinoma coexistent with adenomyosis.

It is important, therefore, for the pathologist to be able to identify carcinoma involving the foci of adenomyosis when assessing the myometrial invasion of endometrial carcinoma. In general, myometrial invasion produces the cancerous nests in an irregular fashion with myometrial reactive changes, such as stromal fibrosis, reduction of smooth muscles and marked inflammatory reaction, predominantly with lymph cells as well as without a surrounding of normal endometrium. On the other hand, when the carcinoma involves the foci of adenomyosis, one frequently finds rounded cancerous nests uniform in size,

Table 5.11. Stage I 5-year survival as a function of myometrial invasion

Series	Year	Superficial (%)	Middle third (%)	Outer third (%)	<half (%)	>half (%)
Corscaden and Tovell	1954	–	–	–	74 (54/73)	41 (23/56)
Gusberg and Yannopoulas	1964	–	–	–	70 (96/137)	34 (94/276)
Climie and Rachminoff	1965	–	–	–	80 (20/25)	56 (23/41)
Cheon	1969	–	–	–	77 (70/91)	42 (31/73)
Austin and MacMahon	1969	–	–	–	95 (239/252)	81 (163/201)
Nison and Koller	1969	–	–	–	89 (205/230)	76 (131/172)
Vongtama et al.	1970	–	–	–	–	65 (19/29)
Sall et al.	1970	92 (75/81)	85 (34/40)	75 (16/21)	–	–
Lewis et al.	1970	88 (36/41)	75 (21/28)	55 (12/22)	–	–
Welander et al.	1972	–	–	–	90 (28/31)	65 (15/23)
Frick et al.	1973	81 (45/56)	85 (23/33)	67 (16/24)	–	–
Keller et al.	1974	–	–	–	87 (36/41)	57 (18/23)
Homesley et al.	1976	–	–	–	84 (254/302)	61 (93/152)
Li	1988	–	–	–	89 (138/155)	52.8 (19/36)

residue of benign endometrial stroma and/or glands on the periphery of the nests, and mild or no lymphatic cell reaction. Involvement of adenomyosis and the depth of true myometrial invasion should be separately commented upon in the pathology report in order to assess prognosis accurately. If the previous diagnosis of myometrial invasion in endometrial carcinoma can be retrospectively reviewed, one will find that the carcinoma involving the foci of adenomyosis is sometimes misdiagnosed as myometrial invasion of endometrial carcinoma.

5.3.5 Cervical Involvement

In 1941, Heyman et al. were the first to recognize the prognostic importance of cervical involvement by endometrial carcinoma. Recent studies reported the 5-year survival to range from 46% to 81.4% (Homesley et al. 1977; Surwit et al. 1978; Bruckman et al. 1978; Gagnon et al. 1979; Prem et al. 1979). Li et al. reported decreasing survival from 77.6% to 59.6% for clinical stage I and II and from 82.2% to 63.6% for surgicopathologic stage I and II, respectively (Li SY 1988) (Table 5.12). Of the 7561 patients involved in 17 individual studies cited by Rutledge, 881 or 11.6% had clinical stage II endometrial carcinomas (Rutledge 1974). The reported incidence ranges from 2.6% to more than 30% (Wade et al. 1967; Prem et al. 1979). Of the 46 consecutive patients with clinical stage II endometrial carcinomas treated at the Mayo Clinic between 1952 and 1973, only 28 were found to have stage II disease at operation. The true-positive rate was 61% and false-positive rate 39% (Wallin et al. 1984). Li et al. (1988) reported a false-positive rate in 37 (or 56.1%) of 66 patients with clinical stage II. The reasons for false-positive results may be: (a) the curettage sample failed to show endocervical glandular involvement; (b) the curettage sample was thought to be from the endocervix, but in fact the tumor was present in the lower uterine segment at pathologic examination, and the endocervix was not involved; and (c) the curettage sample was taken from a false canal which had been polluted by carcinoma (iatrogenic state II).

Table 5.12. Endometrial carcinoma. Five-year survival versus cervical involvement

Stage	Five-year survival (%)
FIGO I	77.6
FIGO II	59.6*
Surgicopathologic I	82.2
Surgicopathologic II	63.6**

* χ^2 test ($P < 0.01$).
**χ^2 test ($P < 0.05$).

Cervical involvement was incorporated in the FIGO staging classification in 1971. Unfortunately, precise histopathologic criteria were not set forth. Currently, stage II classification requires the presence of carcinoma that involves, is contiguous to, or is directly beneath the endocervical glands.

Recent reports have pointed out that stage II endometrial carcinoma should include macroscopic involvement of the cervix (overt group) and microscopic involvement of the cervix (occult group). Several reports showed an 80% 5-year survival for microscopic cervical involvement, and only a 50% 5-year survival for macroscopic involvement. Therefore, the author of this monograph proposed that the difference between them should be considered in designing the treatment. Homesely et al. (1977) reported that the survival was more favorable to endometrial carcinoma with occult rather than overt cervical involvement.

5.3.6 Uterine Size

Uterine size is incorporated into the subgrouping Ia and Ib of FIGO stage I patients, Healy and Brown (1939) suggested the relationship between uterine size and prognosis in endometrial carcinoma, but the real influence of uterine size on prognosis has been controversial. Chen (1985) demonstrated a progressive increase in lymph node metastases with increase in size of the uterus. Lymph node metastases were present in 9 of 67 patients (13.4%) with a uterine cavity smaller than 8 cm and in 9 of 27 patients (33.3%) with a uterine cavity larger than 8 cm. Among the 1761 patients summarized by Jones (1975), there were 1153 with a normal-sized uterus and 578 patients with an enlarged uterus. The 5-year survival was 85.4% in patients with a normal-sized uterus and 66.6% in patients with an enlarged uterus. Jones (1975) supported the idea that the enlarged uterus in endometrial carcinoma infers a worse prognosis.

De Muelenaere (1975) distinguished stages Ia and Ib in 71 patients with stage I endometrial carcinoma using a uterine cavity of 8 cm and a uterine cavity of 10 cm as the criteria. Five-year survival for patients with a cavity smaller than 8 cm was 71.8% (28/39 cases), for patients with a cavity larger than 8 cm it was 81.3% (26/32 cases), for patients with a cavity larger than 10 cm it was 78.2% (43/55 cases), and for patients with a cavity larger than 10 cm it was 68.8% (11/16 cases). Therefore, this author suggested that a uterine cavity of 10 cm is a better criterion for assessing survival. However, Lutz et al. (1978) pointed out that uterine size does not always reflect tumor volume as concomitant benign lesions of the uterus like leiomyomata or adenomyosis may contribute to the enlargement in size of the uterus. There have been several reports suggesting that there is no relationship between uterine size and 5-year survival. In a group of 225 stage I endometrial carcinoma patients reviewed by Nahhas et al. (1971), no relationship between uterine size and 5-year survival was found. Malkasian et al. (1980) found no relationship between uterine size and 5-year survival in 409 patients with endometrial carcinoma. Boronow noted no difference in 5-year survival between patients with stage Ia and Ib endometrial carcinoma, if 5-year survival was also corrected by histologic grade (Boronow 1977).

In view of the previous discussion, it can be stated that the influence of uterine size on the prognosis of endometrial carcinoma remains to be confirmed in further clinical practice.

5.3.7 Histologic Differentiation

Histologic grade is correlated with myometrial invasion and lymph node involvement. Therefore, it has been accepted as a sensitive indicator of prognosis. Creasman et al. (1976) reported a higher percentage of pelvic and paraaortic lymph node involvement with increasing grade. Pelvic lymph node involvement rises from 3%–5.5% in grade I to 26.0%–36.0% in grade III and paraaortic lymph node involvement from 0%–1.5% in grade I to 28.0%–37.5% in grade III (Tables 5.13, 5.14). Boronow et al. (1984) have reported a similar result (Table 5.15).

Table 5.13. Stage I endometrial carcinoma: histologic grade versus status of paraaortic lymph nodes

Series	Grade	Patients (n)	Patients with positive nodes (%)
Piver 1982	G_1	11	0
Creasman et al. 1976		65	1.5
Piver 1982	G_2	22	13.6
Creasman et al. 1976		50	4.0
Piver 1982	G_3	8	37.5
Creasman et al. 1976		25	28.0

Table 5.14. Stage I endometrial carcinoma: histologic grade versus status of pelvic lymph nodes

Series	Grade	Patients (n)	Patients with positive nodes (n)	($\%$)
Lewis et al. 1970	G_1	36	2	5.5
	G_2	50	5	10
	G_3	19	5	26
Creasman et al. 1976	G_1	65	2	3
	G_2	50	5	10
	G_3	25	9	36

Table 5.15. Stage I endometrial carcinoma: histologic grade versus status of pelvic and paraaortic lymph nodes. (Adapted from Boronow et al. 1984)

| | | Patients with positive nodes | |
Grade	Patients (n)	Pelvic nodes (%)	Paraaortic nodes (%)
G_1	93	2.2	1.1
G_2	88	11.4	6.8
G_3	41	26.8	24.4
Total	222	10.4	7.6

5.3.8 Histologic Type

The relationship between histologic type of tumor and survival may also be important. Reagan and Fu (1981) reported that the overall 5-year survival was 72% for patients with endometrial adenocarcinoma, 68% for patients with endometrial adenoacanthoma, but 26% for patients with endometrial adenosquamous carcinoma. Boutselis (1978) reported a 24.3% 5-year survival for endometrial adenosquamous carcinoma and in another report the 5-year survival was 35.3% (Silverberg et al. 1972). Alberhasky et al. (1982) found that the median age at diagnosis was 65 years for patients with endometrial adenosquamous carcinoma, 60 years for adenoacanthoma, and 58 years for adenocarcinoma. The 5-year survival was 87% for adenoacanthoma and 47% for adenosquamous carcinoma. The reasons of the poor survival for adenosquamous carcinoma may be related to the more advanced stage, the poor differentiation of the tumor, the intensive invasion of the squamous cancer, and the older age at diagnosis.

For several decades, reports have appeared in the medical literature contending that there was progressive increase in the number and relative frequency of cancers having an identifiable squamous component. In the 5-year period beginning in 1942, only 15% of the cancers had a readily recognizable squamous component, while in the 5-year period beginning in 1972, this was apparent in 50.9% of the neoplasms. It has been indicated that a small amount of squamous epithelium may be demonstrated in the majority of endometrial carcinomas if the tissue is thoroughly examined (Sommers 1973).

In the FIGO Annual Report (1985), the 5-year survival of 464 cases of adenosquamous carcinoma and clear cell carcinoma in different histologic grades and clinical stages was presented (Table 5.18). The 5-year survival for adenosquamous carcinoma and clear cell carcinoma was lower than that of all the cases of endometrial carcinoma. Prognosis for women with these two types of lesions must be poorer than for others.

In the 25 cases with endometrial papillary adenocarcinoma presented by Weiser et al. (1985), 23 patients were clinical stage I or II. Of the 23 patients with clinical stage I or II, 47% of the patients had deep myometrial invasion, 23% had lymph node metastases, and the 5-year survival was only 68%. It has been shown that this tumor might invade the myometrium and have lymphatic spread early and extensively. Therefore, the tumor has a poorer prognosis.

Baram et al. (1985) reported an increasing percentage of deep myometrial invasion with increasing grade of tumor (Table 5.16).

The FIGO Annual Report (1985) reported 10 097 patients with endometrial carcinoma during the period 1976–1978, with a review of the relationship between clinical stage, histologic grade, and 5-year survival (Table 5.17). There is a persistent relationship between the grade and survival. It is obvious that the less differentiated the tumor, the worse the prognosis.

5.3.9 Tumor Volume

The correlation between primary tumor volume and prognosis was analyzed in 441 patients with endometrial carcinoma by Trotnow et al. in 1978. The larger the tumor volume the worse the prognosis (Table 5.19).

Trotnow et al. suggested that the tumor volume was a better criterion for the assessment of survival as opposed to uterine size. Johnsson in 1979 and Chen in 1985 presented their data concerning primary tumor volume and lymph node metastases. Johnsson noted 16% of the patients with lymph node metastases if the tumor volume was over half the endometrium. Chen observed that the lymph node metastases were 41.2% if the tumor volume was over one-third of the endometrium.

5.3.10 Distance of the Lesion from the Internal Cervical Os

It is well known that involvement of the cervix in endometrial carcinoma infers an increased possibility of lymph node involvement with a worse prognosis. It is,

Table 5.16. Stage I endometrial carcinoma. Histologic grade versus myometrial invasion. (Adapted from Baram et al. (1985)

Grade	< one-third (n)	(%)	> one-third (n)	(%)
G_1	12/103	11.7	8/103	7.8
G_2	8/45	17.8	14/45	31.1
G_3	11/76	14.5	48/76	63.2

Table 5.17. Review of 10097 cases of adenocarcinoma of the endometrial carcinoma, 1976–1978. Five-year survival by histologic grade and stage of disease. (Adapted from FIGO 1985, p. 129)

Histologic grade	Stage I			Stage II		
	Patients treated (*n*)	Five-year (*n*)	survival (%)	Patients treated (*n*)	Five-year (*n*)	survival (%)
Grade 1	3665	2918	79.6	464	298	64.2
Grade 2	2287	1678	73.4	412	249	60.4
Grade 3	866	508	58.7	278	121	43.5
Not graded	1017	738	72.6	198	106	53.5
Total	7835	5842	74.6	1352	774	57.2

Histologic grade	Stage III			Stage IV		
	Patients treated (*n*)	Five-year (*n*)	survival (%)	Patients treated (*n*)	Five-year (*n*)	survival (%)
Grade 1	167	84	50.3	42	8	19.0
Grade 2	159	55	34.6	71	11	15.5
Grade 3	177	38	21.5	120	9	7.5
Not graded	111	22	19.8	63	3	4.8
Total	614	199	32.4	296	31	10.5

Table 5.18. Review of 464 cases of adenosquamous and clear cell carcinoma of the endometrial carcinoma, 1976–1978. Five-year survival by histologic grade and stage of disease. (Adapted from FIGO 1985, p. 129)

Histologic grade	Stage I			Stage II		
	Patients treated (n)	Five-year (n)	survival (%)	Patients treated (n)	Five-year (n)	survival (%)
Grade 1	57	42	73.7	14	6	
Grade 2	80	58	72.5	37	20	54.1
Grade 3	80	53	66.3	28	15	53.6
Not graded	65	46	70.8	16	11	68.8
Total	282	199	70.6	95	52	54.7

Histologic grade	Stage III			Stage IV		
	Patients treated (n)	Five-year (n)	survival (%)	Patients treated (n)	Five-year (n)	survival (%)
Grade 1	8	3		2	0	
Grade 2	10	2		4	1	
Grade 3	16	0	0.0	22	2	9.1
Not graded	16	2	12.5	9	0	
Total	50	7	14.0	37	3	8.1

Table 5.19. Stage I endometrial carcinoma. Five-year survival in relation to tumor volume in the uterine cavity. (Adapted from Trotnow et al. 1978)

Tumor size (cm)	Five year survival (%)
$\leqslant 1$	91.9
$\leqslant 1.5$	78.5
> 1.5	20.6

therefore, logical that with the same grade of differentiation and degree of myometrial invasion the further the lesion is situated from the cervix the better the prognosis should be. Creasman et al. (1976) analyzed the uterine samples after hysterectomy in stage I endometrial cancers and found that 92% of the lesions were localized in the uterine fundus. Involvement of the isthmus also indicates a worse prognosis. Joelsson et al. (1971) suggested that better localization of the lesion within the uterine cavity with preoperative cervicohysteroscopy be optimal to obtain better treatment planning and prognosis.

5.3.11 Pathology of Pericancerous Endometrium

Mori and Silverberg (1984) proposed that when hyperplasia of the pericancerous endometrium is found in the biopsy, curettage, or hysterectomy specimen, the accompanying carcinoma is of a much more favorable type and extent, and survival is significantly better. The 5-year survivals were 83% and 49% for patients with hyperplasia and without hyperplasia respectively. The reason for this correlation is not fully understood, and possible explanations remain to be discussed.

5.3.12 Peritoneal Cytology

A sample of peritoneal fluids or washings should be routinely examined at laparotomy as an adjunct to staging in patients with endometrial carcinoma. A review of the literature shows that the peritoneal fluids or washings were positive in 11%–18% of patients with endometrial carcinoma (Creasman and Rutledge 1971; Yazigi et al. 1983). Creasman et al. (1981) reported that positive cytology was 13.9% in stage I patients; 32% in stage I patients with outer third deeper myometrial invasion; 34% in stage I patients with positive cytology who developed recurrences; as opposed to only 10% in patients with negative cytologic washings. It seems that cytology is a prognostic factor (Table 5.20).

In a group of 93 patients with stage I endometrial carcinoma reported by Yazigi et al. (1983), the peritoneal cytology was positive in 11% of the patients

Table 5.20. Stage I endometrial carcinoma. Histologic grade, depth of invasion, and peritoneal cytologic findings. (Adapted from Creasman et al. 1981)

Grade and myometrial invasion	Patients (n)	Positive cytologic findings	
		(n)	(%)
G_1	74	8	11
G_2	63	15	24
G_3	30	3	10
Endometrial only	72	6	8
Inner third	60	9	15
Mid third	10	3	30
Outer third	25	8	32
Total	167	26	5.5

with stage I disease, and 10% of these cases with positive cytology underwent intraabdominal recurrence and two patients with negative cytology had peritoneal recurrences. However, the high rate of recurrence and worse prognosis in patients with positive cytology have not yet been confirmed in their study. The malignant peritoneal cytology does not seem to be a prognostic indicator in stage I endometrial carcinoma according to this author's observation. Although there is some doubt as to the real influence of positive peritoneal cytology on prognosis, the authors of this monograph still advocate that positive peritoneal cytology should be taken into consideration in the staging and treatment planning of endometrial carcinoma.

5.3.13 Hormone Receptor

Cytosolic estrogen receptor (ERc) was present in 75% of cases of endometrial carcinoma reported in ten individual studies, ranging from 46% to 100% (Grilli et al. 1977; Friberg et al. 1978; Martin et al. 1979; McCarty et al. 1979; Prodi et al. 1979; Soutter et al. 1979; Spona et al. 1979; Young and Ehrlich 1979; Hunter et al. 1980; Ehrlich et al. 1981). Cytosolic progesterone receptor (PRc) was present in 62% of the cases of endometrial carcinoma reported in nine individual studies, ranging from 33% to 89% (MacLaughlin and Richardson 1976; Grilli et al. 1977; Martin et al. 1979; McCarty et al. 1979; Prodi et al. 1979; Spona et al. 1979; Young and Ehrlich 1979; Hunter et al. 1980; Ehrlich et al. 1981). Li and Liu (1984) reported that the frequency of ERc was 47% and the incidence of PRc was 83%. About 33% of the cases of both ERc and PRc were positive. The level as well as the prevalence of ERc and PRc has been found to be proportional to the degree of differentiation of the tumor (McCarty et al. 1979; Hunter et al. 1980;

Ehrlich et al. 1981). There is a tendency toward ERc and PRc to be present more frequently in well-differentiated than in poorly differentiated tumors, and the behavior of receptor-positive tumors seems to be less aggressive (Creasman et al. 1980).

Studies on the relationship between PRc levels and clinical response to progestin therapy have found that ERc and/or PRc positivity seems to be clearly related to a favorable response to treatment. In Li's series, 89.5% of ERc- and/or PRc-positive patients responded to progestin therapy and 14.3% of ERc- and PRc-negative patients responded to progestin therapy (Li et al. 1988). ERc and/or PRc positivity seems to be an index for assessing the response of endometrial carcinoma to progestin therapy.

5.3.14 Treatment Modalities

The optimal treatment of endometrial carcinoma can only be possible provided thorough pretreatment or preoperative assessment of the patients with endometrial carcinoma has been performed. Individualization should be stressed in order to obtain the best results.

FIGO (1985) reported the correlation between 5-year survival and different treatment modalities in 4518 stage I endometrial carcinoma patients between 1976 and 1978 (Table 5.21). The 5-year survival rate for patients treated with surgery was lower than that in patients treated with surgery followed by intravaginal radiation. In a group of patients with endometrial carcinoma studied in the Cancer Institute Hospital, Beijing, 5-year survival was found in 16 or 41% of 31 stage II patients treated with irradiation and in 41 or 70% of 59 stage II patients treated with surgery or surgery combined with irradiation (Table 5.22) (Li 1988).

In general, it appears that patients with stage I or II endometrial carcinoma, treated with surgery or surgery combined with irradiation, may have a better survival.

In 73 stage III endometrial carcinoma patients in the Cancer Institute Hospital, Beijing, it has been found that the 63.6% 5-year survival in patients treated with surgery and adjuvant irradiation differed significantly from the 21% 5-year survival of patients with irradiation alone ($P < 0.01$) (Li 1988) (Table 5.23).

Failure to control local and regional tumor was the major problem in clinical stage III. Surgical eradication of all macroscopic tumor was of major prognostic importance for patients with stage III carcinoma.

The lower 5-year survival for patients with stage IV endometrial carcinoma is indicative of the lack of adequate available treatment for most of these patients. The role of surgery in patients with stage IV endometrial carcinoma is controversial. Aalders et al. (1984b) suggested that the rationale for pelvic treatment in patients with extrapelvic disease should be to improve the patients' chances of being cured with subsequent therapy. Besides, the relief of local symptoms such as vaginal bleeding, discharge, pain, and impending bowel

Table 5.21. Endometrial carcinoma, 1976–1978: 4518 cases of adenocarcinoma stage I, treated with primary surgery alone or followed by irradiation. Five-year survival by grade of differentiation and mode of treatment. (Adapted from FIGO 1985, p. 132)

Mode of treatment	Grade 1			Grade 2		
	Patients treated	Five-year survival (n)	(%)	Patients treated	Five-year survival (n)	(%)
Primary surgery	734	601	81.9	324	253	78.1
Primary surgery + vaginal radium	761	681	89.5	365	322	88.2
Primary surgery + external radium	255	196	76.9	190	139	73.2
Primary surgery + combined vaginal and external radium	524	437	83.4	336	255	75.9
	Grade 3			Not graded		
Primary surgery	114	69	60.5	210	172	81.9
Primary surgery + vaginal radium	94	74	78.7	186	160	86.0
Primary surgery + external radium	106	59	55.7	77	60	77.9
Primary surgery + combined vaginal and external radium	119	72	60.5	123	97	78.9

Table 5.22. Five-year survival and primary treatment modalities in patients with endometrial carcinoma, clinical stage II

Treatment modality	Patients (n)	Five-year survival (n)	(%)
Irradiation	39	16	41
Surgery and/or irradiation	59	41	70*
Total	98	57	58.2

*χ^2 test ($P < 0.05$)

Table 5.23. Five-year survival and primary treatment modalities in patients with endometrial carcinoma, clinical stage III

Treatment modality	Patients (n)	Five-year survival (n)	(%)
Irradiation	62	13	21
Surgery and/or irradiation	11	7	63.6*
Total	73	20	27.4

*χ^2 test ($P<0.01$)

obstruction results in an improvement in the quality of life. As most patients are unsuitable for surgery (73%), radiotherapy will play an important role in the treatment of patients with stage IV endometrial carcinoma.

As mentioned above, there are multiple prognostic factors in each stage of the disease. Pretreatment evaluation of resistance factors in patients and clinico-pathologic entities of tumor require physicians to individualize therapy to obtain the best results and prognosis.

References

Aalders JG, Abeler V, Kolstad P et al. (1980) Post-operative external irradiation and prognostic parameters in stage I endometrial carcinoma: clinical and histopathologic study of 540 patients. Obstet Gynecol 56:419–427

Aalders JG, Abeler V, Kolstad P (1984a) Recurrent adenocarcinoma of the endometrium: a clinical and histopathological study of 379 patients. Gynecol Oncol 17:85–103

Aalders JG, Abeler V, Kolstad P (1984b) Stage IV endometrial carcinoma: a clinical and histopathological study of 83 patients. Gynecol Oncol 17:75–84

Alberhasky RC, Connelly PJ, Christopherson WM (1982) Carcinoma of the endometrium. IV. Mixed adenosquamous carcinoma. Am J Clin Pathol 77:655–664

Austin JH, MacMahon B (1969) Indicators of prognosis in carcinoma of the corpus uteri. Surg Gynecol Obstet 128:1247–1252

Baram A, Figer A, Inbar M et al. (1985) Endometrial carcinoma stage I – comparison of two different treatment regimes – evaluation of risk factors and its influence on prognosis; suggested step by step treatment protocol. Gynecol Oncol 22:294–301

Berman ML, Barlow SC, Lagasse LD et al. (1980) Prognosis and treatment of endometrial cancer. Am J Obstet Gynecol 136:679–688

Boronow RC (1977) Endometrial cancer: staging, pre-treatment evaluation and factors in outcome. In: Gray LA Sr (ed) Endometrial carcinoma and its treatment: the role of irradiation, extent of surgery, and approach to chemotherapy, vol III. Thomas, Springfield, p 38–57

Boronow RC, Morrow CP, Creasman WT et al. (1984) Surgical staging of endometrial cancer: clinical–pathologic findings of a prospective study. Obstet Gynecol 63:825–838

Boutselis JG (1978) Endometrial carcinoma: prognostic factors and treatment. Surg Clin North Am 58:109–119

Bruckman JE, Goodman RL, Murthy A, Marck A (1978) Combined irradiation and surgery in the treatment of stage II carcinoma of the endometrium. Cancer 42:1146–1151

Chen SS (1985) Extrauterine spread in endometrial carcinoma clinically confined to the uterus. Gynecol Oncol 21:23–31

Cheon H (1969) Prognosis of endometrial carcinoma. Obstet Gynecol 34:680–684

Climie ARW, Rachmaninoff N (1965) A ten year experience with endometrial carcinoma. Surg Gynecol Obstet 120:73–78

Connelly PJ, Alberhasky RC, Christopherson WM (1982) Carcinoma of the endometrium III. Analysis of 865 cases of adenocarcinoma and adeno-canthoma. Obstet Gynecol 59:569

Corscaden JA, Tovell HMM (1954) The management of carcinoma of the corpus. Am J Obstet Gynecol 68:737–760

Creasman WT, Rutledge FN (1971) The prognostic value of peritoneal cytology in gynecologic malignant disease. Am J Obstet Gynecol 110:773–781

Creasman WT, Borrow RC, Morrow CP et al. (1976) Adenocarcinoma of the endometrium: its metastatic lymph node potential. A preliminary report. Gynecol Oncol 4:239–243

Creasman WT, McCarty KS, Sr, Barton TK et al. (1980) Clinical correlates of estrogen and progesterone-binding proteins in human endometrial adenocarcinoma. Obstet Gynecol 55:363–370

Creasman WT, DiSaia PJ, Blessing J et al. (1981) Prognostic significance of peritoneal cytology in patients with endometrial cancer and preliminary data concerning therapy with intraperitoneal radiopharmaceuticals. Am J Obstet Gynecol 141:921–929

DeMuelenaere GF (1975) Prognostic factors in endometrial carcinoma. S Afr Med J 49:1695–1698

DiSaia PJ, Creasman WT (1981) Adenocarcinoma of the uterus. In: DiSaia PJ, Creasman WT (eds) Clinical gynecologic oncology. Mosby, St Louis, p 128–151

DeSombre ER, Greene GL, King WT, Jensen EV (1984) Estrogen receptors, antibodies and hormone dependent cancer. In: Gurpide E, Calandra, Levy C, Soto RJ (eds) Hormones and Cancer. Liss, New York, Vol 142 1–21

Ehrlich CE, Young PCM, Cleary RE (1981) Cytoplasmic progesterone and estradiol receptors in normal, hyperplastic, and carcinomatous endometria: therapeutic implications. Am J Obstet Gynecol 141:539–546

Emge LA (1962) The elusive adenomyosis of the uterus. Am J Obstet Gynecol 83:1541–1563

FIGO (1985) Annual report 19:126

Friberg LG, Kullander S, Persijn JP, Korsten CB (1978) On receptors for estrogen (E_2) and androgens (DHT) in human endometrial carcinoma and ovarian tumours. Acat Obstet Gynecol Scand 57:265–271

Frick HC, Munnell EW, Richart RM et al. (1973) Carcinoma of endometrium. Am J Obstet Gynecol 115:663–676

Gagnon JD, Moss WT, Gabourel LS, Stevens KR (1979) External irradiation in the management of stage II endometrial carcinoma. Cancer 44:1247–1251

Giammalvo JT, Kaplan K (1958) The incidence of endometriosis interna in 120 cases of carcinoma of the endometrium. Am J Obstet Gynecol 75:161–166

Greenwood SM (1976) The relation of adenomyosis uteri to coexistent endometrial carcinoma and endometrial hyperplasia. Obstet Gynecol 48:68–72

Grilli S, Ferrari AM, Gola G et al. (1977) Cytoplasmic receptors for 17β-estradiol, 5α-dihydrotestosterone and progesterone in normal and abnormal human uterine tissue. Cancer Lett 2:247–258

Gusberg SB, Yannopoulos D (1964) Therapeutic decision in corpus cancer. Am J Obstet Gynecol 88:157–162

Gusberg SB (1978) Cancer of the endometrium: diagnosis and histogenesis. Corscaden's gynecologic cancer, 5th edn. Williams and Wilkins, Baltimore, p 265–300

Hall JB, Young RH, Nelson JH (1984) The prognostic significance of adenomyosis in endometrial carcinoma. Gynecol Oncol 17:32–40

Hawksworth W (1964) The treatment of carcinoma of the body of the uterus. Proc R Soc Med 57:467–478

Healy WR, Brown RL (1939) Experience with surgical and radiation therapy in carcinoma of the corpus uteri. Am J. Obstet Gynecol 38:1

Hernandez E, Woodruff JD (1980) Endometrial adenocarcinoma arising in adenomyosis. Am J Obstet Gynecol 138:827–832

Homesley HD, Boronow RC, Lewis JL (1976) Treatment of adenocarcinoma of the endometrium at Memorial-James Ewing Hospital 1949–1965. Obstet Gynecol 47:100–105

Homesley HD, Boronow RC, Lewis JL Jr. (1977) Stage II endometrial adenocarcinoma: Memorial Hospital for cancer, 1949–1965. Obstet Gynecol 49:604–608

Hunter RE, Longcope C, Jordon VC (1980) Steroid hormone receptors in adenocarcinoma of the endometrium. Gynecol Oncol 10:152–161

Joelsson, I, Levine RV, Moberger G (1971) Hysteroscopy as an adjunct in determining the extent of carcinoma of the endometrium. Am J Obstet Gynecol 111:696–702

Johnsson JE (1979) Recurrences and metastasis in carcinoma of the uterine body correlated to the size and localization of the primary tumor. Acta Obstet Gynecol Scand 58:405–408

Jones HW (1975) Treatment of adenocarcinoma of the endometrium. Obstet Gynecol Surv 30:147–169

Kauppila A, Grönroos M, Niemineu U (1982) Clinical outcome of endometrial cancer. Obstet Gynecol 60:473–480

Keller D, Kempson RL, Levine G, McLennan C (1974) Management of the patient with early endometrial carcinoma. Cancer 33:1108–1116

Lewis BV, Stallworthy JA, Cowdell R (1970) Adenocarcinoma of the body of the uterus. J Obstet Gynecol Br Commonw 77:343–348

Li SY (1988) Prognosis of endometrial carcinoma. In: Li SY (ed) Endometrial carcinoma. People's Medical Publishing House, Beijing, p 169–198

Li SY, Liu ZM (1984) Estrogen and progesterone receptor in endometrial carcinoma and treatment with 17α-hydroxyprogesterone caproate. J Chin Oncol 6:429–431

Li SY, Wang EY, Li JX et al. (1988) Estrogen receptor and progesterone receptor assay as an index of response to hormone therapy in endometrial cancer. J Practical Oncol 2(4):28–32

Lutz MH, Underwood PB Jr, Kreutner A Jr, Miller MC (1978) Endometrial carcinoma: a new method of classification of therapeutic and prognostic significance. Gynecol Oncol 6:83–94

MacLaughlin DT, Richardson GS (1976) Progesterone binding by normal and abnormal human endometrium. J Clin Endocrinol Metab 42:667–678

Malkasian GD, Annegers JF, Fountain KS (1980) Carcinoma of the endometrium: stage I. Am J Obstet Gynecol 136:872–888

Manetta A, Delgado G, Petrilli E et al. (1986) The significance of paraaortic node status in carcinoma of the cervix and endometrium. Gynecol Oncol 23:284–290

Marcus CC (1962) Relationship of adenomyosis uteri to endometrial hyperplasia and endometrial carcinoma. Am J Obstet Gynecol 82:408–416

Martin PM, Rolland PH, Gammerre M et al. (1979) Estradiol and progesterone receptors, histopathological examinations and clinical responses under progestin therapy. Int J Cancer 23:321–329

Mattingly RF (1977) Malignant tumors of the uterus. Mattingly RF, Thompson J D (eds) In: Telinde's Operative Gynecology, 5th edn. Lippincott, Philadelphia, p 845–876

McCarty KS Jr, Barton TK, Fetter BF et al. (1979) Correlation of estrogen and progesterone receptors with histological differentiation in endometrial adenocarcinoma. Am J pathol 96:171–182

Milton PJD, Metters JS (1972) Endometrial carcinoma – an analysis of 355 patients treated at St Thomas Hospital, 1945–1969. J Obstet Gynecol Br Commonw 79:455

Molitor JJ (1971) Adenomyosis: a clinical and pathological appraisal. Am J Obstet Gynecol 110:275–282

Mori T, Silverberg SG (1984) Endometrial carcinoma: nontumor factors in prognosis. Gynecol Oncol 17:259

Morrow CP, DiSaia PJ, Townsend DE (1973) Current management of endometrial carcinoma. Obstet Gynecol 42:399–408

Morrow CP, Creasman WT, Homesley H et al. (1986) Recurrence in endometrial carcinoma as a function of extended surgical staging data. In: Morrow CP, Smart GE (eds) Gynecological oncology. Springer, Berlin Heidelberg New York, p 147–153

Nahhas WA, Lund CJ, Rudolph JH (1971) Carcinoma of the corpus uterine: a 10-year review of 225 patients. Obstet Gynecol 38:564–570

Ng ABP, Reagan JW (1970) Incidence and prognosis of endometrial carcinoma by histologic grade and extent. Obstet Gynecol 35:437–443

Nilson PA, Koller O (1969) Carcinoma of the endometrium in Norway, 1957–1960, with special reference to treatment results. Am J Obstet Gynecol 105:1099–1109

Nolan JF, Huen A (1976) Prognosis in endometrial cancer. Gynecol Oncol 4:384–390

Ostor AG, Adam R, Gutteridge BH et al. (1982) Endometrial carcinoma in young women. Aust NZ J Obstet Gynecol 22:38–42

Owelabi TO, Stickler RC (1977) Adenomyosis – a neglected diagnosis. Obstet Gynecol 50:424–427

Piver MS, Lele SB, Barlow JJ et al. (1982) Paraaortic lymph node evaluation in stage I endometrial carcinoma. Obstet Gynecol 59:97–100

Plentl AA, Friedman AE (1971) Lymphatic system of the female genitalia. Saunders, Philadelphia, p 135

Prem KA, Adcock LL, Okagaki T, Jones TK (1979) The evolution of a treatment program for adenocarcinoma of the endometrium. Am J Obstet Gynecol 133:803

Prodi G, DeGiovanni C, Galli MC et al. (1979) 17β-Estradiol, 5α-dihydrotestosterone, progesterone and cortisol receptors in normal and neoplastic human endometrium. Tumori 65:241–253

Reagan JW, Fu YS (1981) Pathology of endometrial carcinoma. In: Coppleson M (ed) Gynecologic oncology. Churchill Livingstone, Edinburgh, p. 546–570

Rutledge FN (1974) The role of radical hysterectomy in adenocarcinoma of the endometrium. Gynecol Oncol. 2:331–347

Sall S, Sonnenblick B, Stone ML (1970) Factors affecting survival of patients with endometrial adenocarcinoma. Am J Obstet Gynecol 107:116–123

Silverberg SG, Bolin MG, DeGiorgi LS (1972) Adenoacanthoma and mixed adeno-squamous carcinoma of the endometrium: a clinico-pathological study. Cancer 30:1307–1314

Silverberg SG, Makowski EL (1975) Endometrial carcinoma in young women taking oral contraceptive agents. Obstet Gynecol 46:503–506

Sommers SC (1973) Carcinoma of endometrium. In: Norris JH, Hertig AT, Abell MR (eds) The uterus. Williams and Wilkins, Baltimore, p 276–298

Soutter WP, Hamilton K, Leake RE (1979) High affinity binding of estradiol-17β in the nuclei of human endometrial cells. J Steroid Biochem 10:529–534

Spona J, Ulm R, Bieglmayer C, Husslein P (1979) Hormone serum levels and hormone receptor contents of endometria in women with normal menstrual cycles and patients bearing endometrial carcinoma. Gynecol Obstet Invest 10:71–80

Surwit EA, Fowler WC Jr, Rogoff EE (1978) Stage II carcinoma of the endometrium: an analysis of treatment. Obstet Gynecol 52:97–99

Surwit EA, Joelsson I, Einhorn N (1981) Adjunctive radiation therapy in the management of stage I cancer of the endometrium. Obstet Gynecol 58:590–595

Trotnow S, Becker H, Paterok EM (1978) Tumour volume of endometrial cancer. In: Brush M, Taylor RW (eds) Endometrial cancer. Baillière Tindall, Eastbourne

Vongtama V, Kurohara SS, Badib AO, Webster JH (1970) The value of adjuvant irradiation in the treatment of endometrial carcinoma stage I group 1. Cancer 25:45–49

Wade ME, Kohorn EI, Morris JM (1967) Adenocarcinoma of the endometrium: evaluation of preoperative irradiation and factors influencing prognosis. Am J Obstet Gynecol 99:869–876

Wallin TE, Malkasian GD, Gaffey TA et al. (1984) Stage II cancer of the endometrium: a pathologic and clinical study. Gynecol Oncol 18:1–17

Weed JC, Greary WL, Holland JB (1966) Adenomyosis of the uterus. Clin Obstet Gynecol 9:412–421

Weiser EB, Hoskins WJ, Bibro MC et al. (1985) Papillary adenocarcinoma of the endometrium. Gynecol Oncol 20:249

Welander CA, Griem ML, Newton M, Marks JE (1972) Staging and treatment of endometrial carcinoma. J Reprod Med 8:41–46

Wu BZ, Tang MY, Lang JH (1982) Endometrial carcinoma. In: Lin QZ (ed) Gynecologic oncology. People's Medical Publishing House, Beijing, p 85–104

Yazigi R, Piver MS, Blumenson L (1983) Malignant peritoneal cytology as prognostic indicator in stage I endometrial cancer. Obstet Gynecol 62:359–362

Yoonessi M, Anderson DG, Morley GW (1979) Endometrial carcinoma: causes of death and sites of treatment failure. Cancer 43:1944–1950

Young PCM, Ehrlich CE (1979) Progesterone receptors in human endometrial cancer. In: Thompson EB, Lippman ME (eds) Steroid receptors and the management of cancer, Vol I. CRC Press, Boca Raton, p 135–160

6 Laboratory Research

Recent advances in laboratory research and their clinical application have enabled the clinician to reconcile clinical observations with related scientific observations of which the identification and detection of estrogen and progesterone receptor proteins in the cytosol of endometrial carcinoma have promoted hormone therapy; and it has been possible to estimate the prognosis in patients with endometrial carcinoma. The usefulness of monoclonal antibodies in making early diagnosis, and monitoring treatment and prognosis in patients with ovarian cancer is well demonstrated. Monoclonal antibodies have also been described in endometrial carcinoma. Cell cultures of gynecologic cancers in vivo and in vitro have a long history and have contributed to cytobiologic research of gynecologic neoplasia. In this chapter, an attempt will be made to describe in some detail the current knowledge concerning steroid hormone receptor and monoclonal antibody, which have been studied in patients with gynecologic cancers.

6.1 Steroid Hormone Receptors of Endometrial Carcinoma

Radioimmunoassay was first devised in 1960 by Yalow and Berson to measure minute amounts of insulin in the body by the use of radioiodine-labeled insulin and guinea pig anti-insulin serum. The method was further expanded to measure not only a number of other proteins and peptide but also compounds of low molecular weight such as steroids and pharmaceuticals (haptens). This saturation assay or competitive assay enables a deeper understanding of the interaction between hormones and receptors to be obtained.

There are three types of hormone receptors based on the localization of receptors in cells. For peptide hormones, catecholamines, and releasing factors, specific receptors are on the external surface of the plasma membrane of target tissue cells. For steroid hormones, receptors are found initially in the soluble intracellular compartment of the cell. When the steroid binds, the receptors, modified by the bound hormone, attach to the chromatin of the target tissue cells and are then found predominantly in the nucleus. For thyroid hormones, the intracellular binding sites that best fulfill the criteria for receptors are found in the chromatin of target cells, whether the hormone is present or not.

6.1.1 Discovery of Sex Steroid Hormone Receptors

Jensen and Jacobson from the Ben May Laboratory for Cancer Research, University of Chicago, made a major contribution to the study of hormone action when they synthesized [^{3}H]estradiol ([^{3}H] E$_2$) with a very high specific radioactivity in 1962 (Jensen 1962). By injecting female rats with [^{3}H]E$_2$, Jensen and his colleagues showed that the hormone is retained longer in the uterus than it is in other tissues, e.g., muscle and blood. The uterus is considered a "target" organ of estrogen, whereas muscle and blood are not. This early investigation strongly suggested that some agent had high affinity to hormones in the target cell, binds to the steroid hormones, and prevents their escape; but there is a lack of that agent in nontarget cells, so the hormones may pass through the plasma membrane in both directions and its concentration inside the cell cannot exceed the concentration in the bloodstream.

In 1968, Jenson et al. demonstrated a protein substance called estrogen receptor (ER) in the uterus, vagina, and pituitary, and suggested that receptor-estradiol interactions contain two different phenomena, i.e., uptake and retention. This is the "two-step principle" of receptor-hormone interactions (Jensen et al. 1968). Since then, similar steroid-target organ interactions have been observed for all steroid hormones. In the subsequent research, two important criteria were established for hormone receptors. First, the receptor molecule must be present in the target cells of the hormone but absent in all other cells. Second, the receptor molecule should have a high affinity for its particular hormone but low affinity for other steroids with different biologic activity.

In a series of studies, O'Malley and Schrader found that hormone-receptor complexes were able to bind directly to chromatin isolated from the nucleus; thereby it was revealed that the hormone-receptor complexes can directly bind to the genome to control the synthesis of new protein (O'Malley and Schrader 1976). This mechanism is clearly applicable to the production of hormone-dependent products as in the example of ovalbumin production by the chick oviduct (Baxter and Funder 1979).

Estrogen may stimulate proliferation of the ductal tissue in the breast, the glands and stroma of the endometrium, and the granulosa cells in the ovary. The mitogenic action of estrogen on the normal human endometrium is assessed by finding glandular and stromal mitoses (Noyes et al. 1950). Its action has never been satisfactorily demonstrated in vitro, however, and the possibility exists that its mitogenic action may be indirect (Sonnenschein and Soto 1980a; Sonnenschein and Soto 1980b; Sirbasku et al. 1981). Estrogen receptors of lower affinity that are associated with nucleus (nuclear type II receptors) may be concerned with mitotic events, whereas the high-affinity receptors of the cytosol may not be (Markaverich et al. 1981a; Markaverich et al. 1981b). The presence of receptors that have somehow arrived in the nucleus without their cargo of steroid hormone or have appeared there endogenously suggests that the cells that contain them may be stimulated continuously in the absence of estrogen. Originally demonstrated in cultured breast cancer cells whose growth was estrogen-independent but was blocked by antiestrogens (Zava and McGuire 1977), these receptors have now been found in nonmalignant tissues (Jungblut et al. 1978; Carlsᴄn and Gorski 1980) including normal human endometrium (Fleming and Gurpide 1980; Geier et al. 1980; Levy et al. 1980a).

It is generally agreed that for breast cancer the presence of ER correlates with good prognosis, independent of other prognostic factors such as stage and grade of the tumor, and only tumors that contain ER respond to hormonal manipulation (Consensus Meeting on Steroid Receptors in Breast Cancer 1979). In recent years it has also been found that, for endometrial carcinoma, ER and/or PR positivity seems related to a favorable response to hormonal manipulation (Martin et al. 1979; Benraad et al. 1980; Ehrlich et al. 1981). The behavior of "receptor-positive tumors" seems to be less aggressive (Creasman et al. 1980).

6.1.2 Definition and Characteristics of Steroid Hormone Receptors

All known hormone receptors are protein, which have a molecular weight of about $100\,000-200\,000$ and contain a site or sites to which the hormone may bind. The binding appears to change the confirmation of the receptor, allowing information transfer to the cell, then producing hormone-dependent physiologic phenomena.

Hormone receptors should have the following characteristics:

6.1.2.1 Specificity

Steroid specificity and tissue specificity are included here. Only specific hormone receptors in certain tissues and organs appear to identify the respective hormone or class of hormone, then this binding results in a biologic response, e.g., in male animals, LH was known to act only on Leydig cells and FSH can only combine with Sertoli cells.

6.1.2.2 High Affinity

Steroid receptors are expected to have a high affinity for their respective hormones because the blood levels of steroid are usually $10^{-9}-10^{-10}\,M$. If a tissue is to respond to a hormone via a receptor mechanism in which the hormone binds to the receptor, the receptor must have an affinity for the hormone which is in the range of the blood levels; otherwise no response would occur, e.g., blood concentrations of estradiol (E_2) were $10^{-9}-10^{-10}\,M$, and the dissociation constant (K_d) of estradiol receptor (E_2R) was also $10^{-9}-10^{-10}\,M$.

6.1.2.3 Limited Binding Capacity

The biologic response to a steroid hormone is a saturable phenomenon. If the formation of receptor steroid complexes is obligatory for the biologic response, the steroid receptor concentration should be limited and a specific number of binding sites should be expected. In general, there are 10 000–100 000 receptor-binding sites. This lower binding capacity may easily be saturated by specific ligand. If the binding capacity was changed, the sensitivity and reactivity of target cells to hormones will also be changed. It seems that the changes in binding capacity play an important role in regulating physiologic functions.

6.1.2.4 Reversibility

The relationship between hormones and receptors is a noncovalent binding and the binding rates are dependent on the concentrations of receptors and hormones. The hormone-receptor complexes can also be dissociated at any time. This reversibility of binding may prevent the undue influence of hormones.

6.1.2.5 Correlation with Biologic Response

The hormone-receptor complexes should be demonstrated in vivo with relation to certain physiologic function, otherwise these binding proteins should not be considered as receptors.

6.1.3 Intracellular Mechanism of Action of Steroid Receptors

It is virtually certain that most steroid hormones act on their respective target tissues by the following mechanisms:

6.1.3.1 Lipophilic Characters

According to their lipophilic characters, steroid hormones appear to enter the cells by passive diffusion and readily penetrate through the cell membrane to interact with a cytoplasmic receptor protein. In the cytoplasm, the hormone binds specifically to their receptor within 5–15 s. This binding is a non-covalent binding without consuming energy.

6.1.3.2 Cytoplasmic Receptor-Hormone Complex

The cytoplasmic receptor-hormone (RcS) complex is translocated to the nucleus. Before it is translocated, it undergoes a temperature-dependent transformation step, e.g., molecular weight of receptor and sedimentary coefficient. The transformed receptor is called the nuclear receptor (Rn) because it is able to bind to the nucleus. Jensen et al. (1979) were able to demonstrate the migration of the receptor from the cytoplasm to the nucleus where the hormone-receptor complex (RnS) binds to chromatin, inducing the transcription of specific RNAs via interaction with the genome.

This translocated process involves an energy-requiring activation step, which needs 5–30 min and is probably physiologically irreversible. The retention of RnS in nuclei appears to be an important function in producing physiologic activities.

Anderson et al. suggested that the presence of RnS in the nuclear fraction for approximately 6 h is a requisite for the induction of long-term uterotrophic response. The differential liability of receptor estradiol and receptor estriol complexes was employed. Nuclear receptor estradiol and receptor estriol are equivalent between 1 and 3 h after estrogen injection. Early responses such as increases in wet weight were also equivalent. However, 6 h after injection, receptor estradiol remains significantly higher than receptor estriol, which declines to the level of saline-injected controls. In a corresponding manner, estradiol induced long-term uterotrophic responses, whereas estriol was incapable of such induction (Anderson et al. 1972).

6.1.3.3 Activated Receptor Hormone Complex

The activated receptor hormone complex binds to an "acceptor" site on the chromatin. The steroid probably changes the conformation of the receptor so that a nuclear-binding site on the receptor is exposed. In vivo, activation probably occurs rapidly after the steroid binding and probably does not delay the nuclear-binding reaction. Chromatin consists of DNA and the proteins that package DNA and control its transcription and replication. Chromatin also contains sites (acceptors) for binding the activated steroid-receptor complexes. The DNA of chromatin is important for acceptor activity, but the chromatin proteins seem also to participate in this process. This binding was of rather higher affinity, e.g., E_2R, with a dissociation constant of approximately 10^{-10} M.

6.1.3.4 Chromatin Binding

Chromatin binding activates the transcription of DNA into protein-synthesizing message RNA. The binding of receptor-steroid complexes with the nuclear chromatin results in changes in the levels of specific mRNAs. The response has been selective, in that only a few specific mRNAs are affected by the steroid. The steroid-regulated effects on mRNA levels appear to be due to the action on transcription of the DNA into RNA; this is probably the primary event in most cases. mRNA serves as a template for the construction of a protein. The scheme for steroid hormone action is depicted in Fig. 6.1.

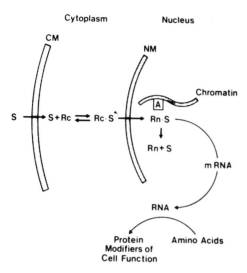

Fig. 6.1. Proposed mechanism of hormone action. *S*, steroid hormone; *Rc*, cytoplasmic receptor; *S*, activated receptor; *CM*, cell membrane; *NM*, nuclear membrane; *Rn*, nuclear translocated receptor; *A*, acceptor site; *mRNA*, messenger RNA

During the past 20 years, considerable effort has been devoted to the elucidation of the molecular mechanism by which steroid hormones regulate gene expression, growth, and function in hormone-responsive cells. However, despite this effort, obscurity and controversy surround most of the processes involved in steroid uptake and binding to appropriate receptor proteins, as well as virtually all of the cellular interactions of steroid receptor complexes, including activation, binding to chromatin, synthesis and degradation of receptor, and the events involved in transcriptional modulation.

Also unclear is the intracellular location of the "extranuclear" unoccupied receptor found in the cytosol of tissue homogenates. Recent biochemical and immunocytochemical data suggest that the majority of functional ER may reside in the nucleus regardless of hormone status, and the binding of hormone to receptor leads to a tighter association of steroid-receptor complex with nuclear components (Welshous et al. 1984; King and Greene 1984; Press and Greene 1984; Press et al. 1985). Welshous et al. (1984) observed that cytochalasin-induced enucleation of rat pituitary (CH3) cells leads to partitioning of unoccupied ER almost exclusively into the nucleoplast fraction; at least 85% of ER were nuclear. The finding that ER is predominantly nuclear, whether or not it is bound to the steroid, contradicts a large body of evidence which has been interpreted to indicate that the free ER is a cytoplasmic protein. There have been several reports in the literature which are comparable with Welshons' findings. These include autoradiographic localization of most of the hormone bindings to the nucleus in "nontranslocation" conditions (Sheridan et al. 1980). The appearance of 4S "cytoplasmic" receptor in the nuclei of some tissues before 5S (nuclear forms which appear after binding of the hormone) and evidence that some estrogens produce full physiologic effects were noticed even though the receptor appears entirely in the cytosol extracts of homogenized cells. A recent immuno-

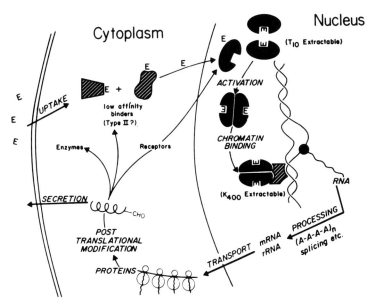

Fig. 6.2. Revised schematic diagram of estrogen action in a target cell. (Reproduced from DeSombre et al. 1984)

cytochemical study indicated that antibodies to the ER interact only with the nuclei of human endometrium or human mammary tumor cells, whether or not estrogen is present (King and Greene 1984).

   These observations suggested that the majority of unoccupied receptors may actually reside in the nucleus rather than in the cytoplasm as previously thought. This revised interpretation of steroid hormone action is shown schematically in Fig. 6.2. According to this model, the steroid passes through the cell to the nucleus, either unaided or perhaps bound loosely to low-affinity sites in the cytoplasm, where it interacts with unoccupied receptor in the nucleus, resulting in the formation of activated steroid-receptor complex, which becomes more tightly associated with chromatin.

6.1.4 Methodology of Steroid Hormone Receptor Detection

Steroid receptor (SR) determination in making therapeutic decisions has been widely used for breast cancer and for other target tissues under investigation. Therefore, the methods of steroid receptor detection have aroused the interest of all. At present, in the SR determination methods, there are major problems, such as, the specificity of high-affinity/low-affinity binding sites and the specificity of antigenic sites; the accessibility of free/bound receptor and the heterogeneous distribution of receptors in the tissues. Most of the biochemical assays and morphologic methods rely on the steroid-binding properties of receptors. Recently, specific monoclonal antibodies against ER have been prepared, permitting the development of ER enzyme immunoassays (ER-EIAs) and ER immunocytochemical assays (ER-ICAs) which are based on the characteristics of the ER antigenic site rather than the steroid-binding sites determined with other methods. The principles of the various methods of receptor determination are briefly reviewed.

6.1.4.1 Biochemical Methods (Radioligand-Binding Assays)

These methods are the first accurate techniques and are still performed routinely (Martin et al. 1978 a, b 1979). They are based on the detection of radioactive tracers such as tritiated steroid, which makes possible determination of binding constants, binding site concentrations, and specificity of each binding system, i.e., specific and nonspecific system, high-affinity type I system (saturation estradiol concentrations $< 10^{-9}$ M), and low-affinity type II and type III system (saturation estradiol concentrations $> 10^{-9}$ M).

These methods are quantitative, accurate, and reliable. They include dextran-coated charcoal assay (DCC), sucrose density gradient centrifugation (SDG), agar gel electrophoresis, absorption of the receptor onto hydroxylapatite (HAP) or diethylaminoethanol (DEAE) filters, and isoelectric focusing in polyacrylamide gel. The principle of biochemical methods is based on the combined dynamics of hormone and receptor interaction, which is briefly introduced as follows:

6.1.4.1.1 Basic Theory

The interaction between hormone and specific receptor on target cells is a reversible reaction, i.e., hormones may continually bind to receptors, forming hormone-receptor complexes which, on the contrary, may continually dissociate into free hormones and free receptors. This reaction follows the law of mass action.

$$[H] + [R] \underset{K_2}{\overset{K_1}{\rightleftharpoons}} [HR]$$

$[H]$ = hormone concentration K_1 = association constant
$[R]$ = receptor concentration K_2 = dissociation constant
$[HR]$ = hormone-receptor complex concentration

The amount forming hormone-receptor complexes at unit time $= K_1 [H] [R]$

The amount of dissociation from hormone-receptor complexes at unit time $= K_2 [HR]$ when the equilibrium is achieved in the reversible reaction,

$$K_1[H] [R] = K_2[HR]$$

The dissociation constant for the HR complex is defined:

$$K_d = \frac{K_2}{K_1} = \frac{[H]\,[R]}{[HR]}$$

If 50% of the receptors are bound by hormones, i.e., $[H]=[R]$, $[R]=[HR]$, $K_d=[H]$ and when 50% of the receptors are saturated, the free hormone concentrations might be equal to the value of K_d. The lower the value of K_d the higher the affinity. The affinity or association constant (K_a) or its reciprocal of the dissociation constant (K_d) may also act as a parameter of interaction between the hormones and receptors. In general, the value of K_d can be used in the receptor assay and the value of K_a in radioimmunoassay.

6.1.4.1.2 Saturation Analysis

This is usually accomplished by exposing the constant concentration of homogenates of target cells to various concentrations of labeled steroid under equilibrium conditions. When the equilibrium is achieved in the reversible reaction, the amount of labeled steroid-receptor complexes will be measured. It was found that the higher the concentration of labeled steroids the more the labeled steroid-receptor complexes will be formed. Once all receptor-binding sites are occupied by labeled steroid, the amount of labeled steroid-receptor complexes will not increase with the increased amount of labeled steroids. This saturation value represented the highest binding capacity of steroid receptors. If the concentration of labeled steroid hormones is used as an abscissa and the amount of steroid-receptor complexes as an ordinate, the saturation lines will be drawn.

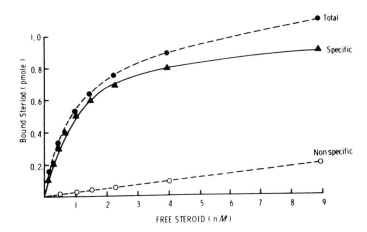

Fig. 6.3. Steroid binding to specific and nonspecific sites. Quantity of specifically bound steroid (▲) is determined by subtracting nonspecific (○) from total binding (●)

The line designated as total in Fig. 6.3 represents the amount of steroid which is bound to the receptor sites and nonspecific binding sites, thus containing both saturable and nonsaturable components. Under practical conditions, in order to define the saturable or receptor component, nonspecific binding sites are measured as the [³H] steroid bound in the presence of a 100-fold molar excess of an unlabeled competitive ligand. The competing nonlabeled steroid will occupy essentially all high-affinity receptor-binding sites but will not interfere appreciably with the binding of [³H] steroid to low affinity, non-specific, or nonsaturable sites. It is assumed that nonspecific binding sites are of low affinity and high capacity relative to the receptor system.

The quantity of specifically bound steroid is determined by subtracting nonspecific from total binding.

For the simplest system, $[H]+[R]\rightleftharpoons[HR]$

where the dissociation constant for the HR complex is defined

$$K_d = \frac{[H][R]}{[HR]} \tag{1}$$

If the free hormone $[F]=[H]$ $\qquad$ (2)
the binding hormone receptor $[B]=[HR]$ $\qquad$ (3)
all the receptor-binding sites $[N]=$ free receptor $[R]$
+ hormone-receptor complexes $[B]$
$[R]=[N]-[B]$ $\qquad$ (4)

Equation 1 then becomes:

$$K_d = \frac{[F][N-B]}{[B]} = \frac{[F][N]}{[B]} - [F]$$
$$K_d + [F] = \frac{[F][N]}{[B]}$$
$$[B] = \frac{[N][F]}{K_d + [F]} \tag{5}$$

When 50% of the receptor sites were occupied with labeled hormones, that is:

$$[B] = \frac{[N]}{2} = \frac{[N][F]}{K_d + [F]}$$
$$K_d = 2[F] - [F] = [F]$$

Under the circumstance of interactions of labeled hormone with receptor, the quantity of labeled hormone is great with respect to the specific binding sites. The difference in concentration between the labeled hormone and specific binding sites is about 100-fold, i.e., $[F]=[H] \therefore K_d=[H]$. Therefore, the dissociation constant may be determined by the concentration of labeled hormones when 50% of the receptor sites were saturated. In general, pM or nM is the calculating unit.

It may be seen from the saturation curves that if the straight line is drawn from the saturation point of the specific binding to the ordinate, the intercept is regarded as the amount of receptor binding at the concentration of tissue homogenates. fM/mg protein is the calculating unit.

6.1.4.1.3 Interpretation of Saturation Parameters with Scatchard Analysis

The principle of Scatchard analysis is as follows:

$$[B] = \frac{[N][F]}{K_d + [F]} \tag{5}$$

$$\frac{1}{[B]} = \frac{K_d + [F]}{[N][F]}$$

$$\frac{1}{B} = \frac{K_d}{[F][N]} + \frac{1}{[N]}$$

Multiplying the equation by $[N][B]$:

$$\frac{[N][B]}{[B]} = \frac{[N][B]K_d}{[F][N]} + \frac{[N][B]}{[N]}$$

$$[N] = \frac{[B]K_d}{[F]} + [B]$$

$$\frac{[B]}{[F]} = \frac{[N] - [B]}{K_d}$$

$$\frac{[B]}{[F]} = -\frac{1}{K_d}[B] + \frac{[N]}{K_d}$$

If the typical data of a binding system that contains only one receptor and linear nonspecific binding are used for Scatchard analysis, the straight line may be obtained (Fig. 6.4) (Scatchard 1949). The affinity or association constant (k_a), or its reciprocal, the dissociation constant (K_d), and the number of receptor sites at saturation (n) may be obtained from the Scatchard plot. The Y-intercept of the Scatchard plot is equal to nK_a or n/K_d. The line is used to extrapolate a point on the abscissa which overestimates the true value of n.

6.1.4.1.4 Measurement of Estrogen and Progesterone Receptors

Measurement of cytosol estrogen receptors (ERc) and progesterone receptors (PRc) was carried out with modified single-point dextran-coated charcoal assay (DCC) in the Cancer Hospital, Beijing (King 1979; Liu 1981; Zhang et al. 1983).

Chemicals and Solvents
Tritiated steroids, (2,4,6,7-^{3}H) 17β-estradiol (^{3}H-E$_2$), specific activity 90–115. Ci/mM, and (6,7-^{3}H) progesterone (4-pregnene-3, 20 dione) (^{3}H-P), specific

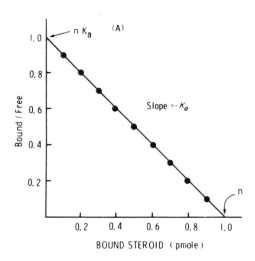

Fig. 6.4. Determination of receptor-binding parameters

activity 55 Ci/mM, as well as unlabeled steroids were obtained from New England Nuclear Corporation. Dextran T-70 was obtained from Pharmacia Fine Chemicals, Inc., and all other chemicals used were of reagent grade and obtained from commercial sources.

1. 100 nM 2,4,6,7-^{3}H 17β-E$_2$
2. 200 nM 6,7-^{3}HP
3. 10 μM stilbestrol
4. 10 μM cortisol
5. 10 μM progesterone
6. Tris-EDTA-DTT (TED) buffer used for ERc assay: 10 mM Tris-HCl, 1.5 mM ethylenediaminetetraacetic acid (EDTA), 1 mM dithiothreitol, 3 mM sodium azide, pH 7.4 at 4°C
7. Tris-EDTA-glyceral-DTT (TEGD) buffer used for PRC assay: 10 mM Tris-HCl, 1.5 mM EDTA, 3 mM sodium azide, 1 mM dithiothreitol, 30% glycerol, pH 7.4 at 4°C
8. Dextran-coated charcoal suspension: 0.5% charcoal, 0.05% dextran T-70 in 0.1% gelatin
9. Scintillation fluid: POPOP 0.5 g, PPO 5 g in 1000 ml toluene

Assay Procedure
All analytic procedures were carried out at 0°–4°C.

Cytosol Preparation.   A quantity of 0.1–0.5 g frozen tissue was weighed and cut into small pieces which were thawed and washed repeatedly with ice-cold TEGD buffer. After mincing, the tissue was suspended in TEGD buffer. The ratio of tissue (W) to buffer (V) was 1:5. The tissue was homogenized with a Brinkman polytron at a power setting of 3.5 in two 10-s bursts with a 2-min cooling interval in iced water between bursts. The homogenate was then centrifuged at 4°C for 30 min at 800 g to yield a cytosol-rich supernatant.

Cytosol Estrogen Receptor (ERc) Assay. Duplicate 200-μl aliquots of cytosol were incubated with 10 μl 100 nM ^{3}H-E$_2$ or 10 μl of 100 nM ^{3}H-E$_2$ and 10 μl 10 μM stilbestrol. The final concentrations of ^{3}H-E$_2$ and stilbestrol in tubes are 5 nM and 0.5 μM respectively. The tubes were incubated for 8–16 h at 4°C. Following the incubation, 200 μl DCC suspension was added to remove the unbound steroids. DCC was removed by centrifugation at 800 g for 10 min at 0°–4°C after being vortexed for 15–30 min and allowed to stand for 10 min. A 150 μl aliquot of the supernatant was then added to 1 ml scintillation cocktail and counted after standing for 12 h.

Cytosol Progesterone Receptor (PRc) Assay. Duplicate 200-μl aliquots of cytosol were incubated with 10 μl 200 nM [^{3}H]P, 10 μl 10 μM cortisol or 10 μl 200 nM [^{3}H]P, 10 μl 10 μM cortisol, and 10 μl 10 μM progesterone. The final concentrations of [^{3}H]P, cortisol, and progesterone in the tubes were 5 nM, 0.5 μM, and 0.5 μM respectively.

The tubes were incubated for 2 h at 0°C. Following the incubation, 200 μl DCC suspension was added to remove the unbound steroids. The DCC was removed by centrifugation at 800 g for 10 min at 0°C after being vortexed for 5 min and allowed to stand for 10 min. A 150-μl aliquot of the supernatant was then added to 1 ml scintillation cocktail and counted after standing for 12 h.

Protein Concentration Assay. Protein concentration was quantitated with the method of Lowry et al. (Lowry et al. 1951).

Calculation. The specific binding was calculated by subtracting the nonspecific binding from the total binding. The receptor unit was represented by fM/mg protein. Specific binding = total binding − nonspecific binding. Although biochemical methods are accurate and reliable, they are not devoid of drawbacks:

1. Endometrial curettings that contain carcinoma may also contain variable amounts of normal or hyperplastic tissue (Horwitz et al. 1981). Because the volume of tissue is limited, most of it should be sent for pathologic examination, leaving only a small amount available for receptor assay. Under these conditions, it may be possible to perform only a single-point saturation assay and risk confusion between high- and low-affinity (type I and type II) receptors.
2. Histologic control of samples is imperative, insuring the tissue analyzed is representative. Pathologists from different institutions are apt to apply somewhat different criteria to distinguish between atypical hyperplasia of the endometrium and cancer of the endometrium and there is unquestionably a great deal of variation between reports from different centers. It is important to have strict pathologic criteria in order to give an accurate assessment. An

example of what might be done in the case of endometrial carcinoma is the report by Robboy and Bradley (1979), who assessed 17 histologic variables: (a) histologic type of tumor; (b) grade; (c) depth of invasion; (d) percentage of squamous component; (e) intracellular and extracellular mucin; (f) presence of ciliated cells; (g) growth pattern (tubular, papillary, solid, and mixed); (h) intercellular bridge; (i) individual cell keratinization; (j) strains composed of squamous cells; (k) intraluminal cellular buds; (l) cytoplasmic eosinophilials ("pink cells"); (m) glycogen content; (n) foam cells in stroma; (o) tumor necrosis; (p) mitotic index; and (q) cyclic phase of adjacent benign endometrium. Six microscopic patterns of tumor have been identified: adenocarcinoma, adenoacanthoma, atypical adenoacanthoma, adenosquamous carcinoma, clear cell adenocarcinoma, and undifferentiated carcinoma. Histologic assessment of ovarian cancer is far more complicated and there are many more problems in tumor sampling.

3. Strict quality control of these methods is needed in order to compare the experimental results between various laboratories.
4. Only unoccupied receptors can be detected. Chamness et al. (1980) reported that only free ERc could be detected if incubated for 18 h at 4°C.
5. Only an average value of receptor concentration from tissue homogenates could be obtained, which do not represent cell heterogeneity in tissue.
6. These methods are expensive, needing sophisticated equipment, and are time consuming to perform.

6.1.4.2 Morphologic Methods

These methods are performed on tissue sections or entire cells, providing information about SR distribution within cells and tissues. Four methods are described here:

6.1.4.2.1 Autoradiography (Edwards et al. 1980; Sheridan et al. 1980; Martin and Sheridan 1982)

This method permits the specific detection of high-affinity binding sites and is a qualitative method allowing tissue structure preservation. It enables SR distribution analysis to be carried out in tissue sections or entire cells. However, even though it has specificity and sensitivity, this method is inappropriate for widespread clinical use due to the following drawbacks:

1. Radiolabeled ligands such as 10^{-9}–10^{-10} M estradiol or analog concentration need long exposure time of over 8 weeks at low temperature ($-40°C$)
2. Diffusion of radiolabeled tracers may occur during the required preincubation.
3. Tissue sections cannot be fixed since fixators extract labeled steroids.

6.1.4.2.2 Histochemical Method Using Spontaneously Fluorescent Steroids (Martin et al. 1978a, b 1983)

This method is based on the spontaneously fluorescent properties of compounds that have a certain affinity for ER. With conventional fluorescent techniques, these compounds can be detected when high concentrations, 10^{-5}–10^{-7} M, are used. However, using a fluorescence microscope equipped with a microchannel image intensifier and a videocamera detector, providing a sensitivity enhancement of 10^4 M, low concentrations, down to 10^{-9} M, can be detected in the cell nucleus, as with autoradiography. This method is, therefore, suitable and convenient for the visualization of high-affinity binding sites and may be applied to tissue section and also to living cells in the cultures. However, the major problem of the method consists of the availability and cost of a video intensification magnifier system.

6.1.4.2.3 Histochemical Method Using Bipolar Tracers (Dandliker et al. 1978; Lee 1978; Barrows et al. 1980)

This method uses steroids conjugated either directly or through bovine serum albumin (BSA) to fluorescein or peroxidase. Although it is easy to perform, it is not suitable for high-affinity binding site detection since high concentrations (10^{-6} M) of labeled estradiol are required, indicating that low-affinity binding sites are more likely detected (Chamness et al. 1980).

6.1.4.2.4 Immunohistochemical Methods Using Antisteroid Antibodies (Nenci et al. 1976; Kurzon and Sternberger 1978; Pertschuk et al. 1978)

These methods first require an incubation with steroid or polyestradiol phosphate and then detection of estradiol bound to antisteroid antibody. Either labeled antisteroid antibodies (fluorescence or peroxidase conjugated) or unlabeled antibody with peroxidase, antiperoxidase (PAP), or avidin biotin peroxidase complex (ABC) can be used. Although these methods are readily applicable to tissue sections, they present two major problems:

1. A high concentration of estradiol (10^{-7} M) is used for the preincubation step, and the low-affinity binding site can be detected.
2. Specificity of antibodies is questionable, particularly when antibodies are diluted to $1/10$–$1/50$.

6.1.4.3 Monoclonal Antireceptor Antibody Assays

New approaches for steroid receptor detection, which are based on monoclonal antibodies to human tumor ER produced by Greene et al. (1980a, b), use the direct antigenic recognition of the receptor molecules. The antibodies recognize the ER independent of the presence or absence of estradiol in the binding sites. The new assays are the solid-phase enzyme immunoassay (EIA) and immuno-cytochemical assay (ICA). Using determination of estrogen receptor as an example, the principle of measurement is described as follows:

6.1.4.3.1 Monoclonal Enzyme Immunoassay of Estrogen Receptors (ER–EIA)

The ER–EIA is based on a "Sandwich" technique. Tumor cytosols are incubated with beads coated with anti-ER monoclonal antibody. During this time, the receptors are immobilized by binding to the antibody, and unbound materials are then removed by aspiration and washing of the beads. A second ER-specific monoclonal antibody conjugated to horseradish peroxidase is added and a complex of layered antibodies and receptors is formed. The addition of enzyme substrate solution (hydrogen peroxide and O-phenylene-diamine-2 HCL) pro-duces a color reaction, the intensity of which is proportional to the amount of receptor present. The receptor level is determined from a standard curve of ER run with the tumor cytosols. Diagrammatic representation of ER-EIA assay is presented in Fig. 6.5.

A multicenter trial was conducted in Europe and the United States under the auspices of Abbott laboratories to determine the reproducibility of ER-EIA and to compare ER levels in a series of locally prepared human breast cancer cytosols as determined by ER-EIA and ER assay currently in use in the participating laboratory (DCC assays in ten laboratories, isoelectrofocusing in one laborat-ory). The data reported on a large series of breast cancer specimens plotted so that linear correlation coefficients and slope could be calculated. The linear correlation coefficients were excellent and the intercepts were in the same range and were not statistically different from O. Each of the slopes was greater than 1, which suggests that ER-EIA may be able to detect receptor proteins that are not measured by the steroid-binding assays. The reproducibility of ER-EIA (inter-assay coefficient of variation, 6%; interlaboratory coefficient of variation, 11% –19%) was somewhat better than that of the DCC method (interlaboratory coefficient of variation, 12%–32%) (Leclercq et al. 1986; Jordan et al. 1986). ER-EIA is a highly sensitive assay which allows ER determination on fine-needle aspirates, the sensitivity of which has been clearly demonstrated for surgical samples. The assay is reliable at cytosol protein concentrations as low as 0.2 mg/ml (1.5 mg/ml for routine steroid-binding assays) (Magdelenat et al. 1986). The ER-EIA method for the determination of ER in high salt extracts of crude nuclear pellets from breast cancer biopsies is a simple and rapid assay for ERn. Total ER is measured, i.e., no distinction is made between hormone-bound ER and free ERn. The values obtained using ER-EIA are about two to threefold higher than those obtained using the HPA (hydroxylapatite) method. The ER-EIA is, therefore, well suited for the routine analysis of ERn in human breast cancer biopsies (Thorpe et al. 1986).

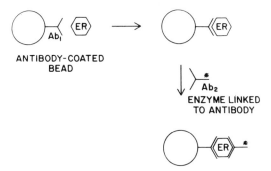

Fig. 6.5. Diagrammatic representation of the ER-EIA bead assay for the determination of ER in breast tumor cytosols. *Ab*, antibody

Nicholson et al. (1986) reported that ER-EIA has been evaluated in 70 human breast carcinomas against a routine cytoplasmic [^{3}H]estradiol-binding assay (ERU). ERU gave a lower number of estrogen receptor-positive tumors (50 out of 70) than did the ER-EIA assay (59 out of 70). The characteristics of the two assays may explain the above results. The routine binding assay was carried out under conditions which measure only the unoccupied receptor sites, whereas the ER-EIA measures both the occupied and unoccupied receptors. Thus, under conditions of occupancy of the steroid-binding sites by endogenous estrogens, ERU would underestimate the true value of ER. Magdelenat et al. (1986) reported the correlation between the ER-EIA and DCC methods on 61 unselected samples of malignant mammary cells. Quantitative correlation between the ER-EIA and DCC methods was high ($r = 0.86$) and the highest ($r = 0.97$) when samples from 13 patients undergoing tamoxifen treatment were excluded. Major discrepancies between the ER-EIA and DCC methods appeared in the patients undergoing tamoxifen therapy and much higher values were obtained by ER-EIA. Eight of the 13 patients were ER negative by DCC but ER positive by ER-EIA. Preliminary observations indicate that in vivo ER modulation by hormones and antihormones should be reevaluated (Magdelenat et al. 1986).

6.1.4.3.2 Monoclonal Enzyme Immunocytochemical Assay and Monoclonal Enzyme Immunohistochemical Assay of Estrogen Receptors (ER-EICA, ER-EIHA)

McClelland et al. used an immunoperoxidase technique utilizing a monoclonal antibody to ER to identify immunoreactive ER in breast carcinoma and examined the relationship between the immunoreactive ER and response to therapy in patients with advanced breast carcinoma. Fifty-six patients were found to be assessable for response to endocrine therapy. Twenty-two patients showed an objective response to some form of endocrine manipulation, and all these had positively stained carcinomas. None of the 17 patients with negatively stained carcinomas responded to endocrine therapy. The relative overall predictive abilities of ER-EICA and DCC techniques showed that ER-EICA correctly classified, i.e., responding ER positive or non-responding ER negataves, 47 of 56 (83.9%) and the DCC 41 of 56 (73.2%). It appears that ER-EICA can predict the outcome of hormone therapy better than DCC in patients with breast carcinoma (McClelland et al. 1986). A monoclonal antibody to human ER protein (H 222 Spr), amplified via immunoperoxidase techniques, was used in the analysis of ER in 452 breast carcinomas and 100 endometrial carcinomas. Immunohistochemical evaluation incorporated both intensity and distribution of staining (HSCORE). Quantitative ER content was determined by DCC analysis and sucrose density gradient analysis. In all cases, H 222 Spr was localized in the nucleus of the target cells. The sensitivities and specificities for HSCORE as compared with the biochemical assays ranged from 80% to 95% and from 74% to 94% respectively. HSCORE correlated with tumor grade of breast and endometrial carcinoma. The data suggest that immunohistochemical receptor localization provides information complementary to standard biochemical assays in the tissues studied (McCarty et al. 1986). DeSombre et al. observed the prognostic usefulness of ER-EICA for human breast cancers of postmenopausal patients and found that positive or negative ER-EICA as well as ER-EICA staining intensity and proportion of ER-EICA-stained cancer cells might relate to patient disease-free interval and survival, independent of patient lymph node involvement (DeSombre et al. 1986). Charpin et al. reported that, when immunohistochemical staining was correlated to biochemical assay, there was an 88% correlation and staining intensity and percentage of positive cells increased significantly ($P < 0.01$) with cytosolic ER levels and were independent of cellularity (Charpin et al. 1986). It was suggested that ER-EIHA and ER-EICA are able to identify biologically significant ER protein because excellent correlation with clinical response was obtained in an initial small cohort of patients (McCarty et al. 1985). The ability to assess heterogeneity of receptor expression, whether between normal elements and tumor or between tumor cells, has considerable potential in furthering an understanding of tumor behavior. In the case of endometrial carcinoma, the ability consistently to separate out malignant components from normal or benign components for the first time allows one to determine more effectively whether the presence of ER can have prognostic implications similar to those of breast carcinoma (McGuire et al. 1975; Byar et al. 1979; Furmanski et al. 1980; Singhakowinta et al. 1980). The identification of substantial portions of tumor that are receptor negative appears to have clinical implications. It may account for at least some of the so-called "biologic false-positives" seen with biochemical assays. The observation of heterogeneous staining in both endometrial carcinoma and breast carcinoma in contrast to relatively homogeneous staining of benign epithelium, myometrium, and uterine stroma raises the question of whether this heterogeneous staining, which reflects a polyclonal tumor, is due to the asynchrony of receptor expression under various physiologic conditions.

However, whatever the degree of improvement of the immunocytochemical assay analysis by the computerized system for image analysis of microscopic preparations may be, it is too early to suggest that ER-EICA could replace ER biochemical quantitative assays since no accurate data for hormone therapy decision and prognosis evaluation are thus far available for ER-EICA. Combined ER analysis in tumor by both binding assays and ER-EICA could improve the predictability of response to hormone therapy.

Although biochemical methods have some drawbacks, it is difficult to replace them by ER-EIHA and ER-EICA.

1. The biochemical methods, e.g., DCC assay, may be used to measure occupied and unoccupied sites in various subcellular components to detect receptor affinity to hormones. Therefore, one should be able to use this procedure in relating receptor occupancy to hormone-induced responses.
2. The majority of published papers on ER and PR status used biochemical assays. Although there is good correlation between ER-EIHA, ER-EICA, and DCC assays, one should be very careful in replacing DCC assay by ER-EIHA or ER-EICA.
3. The cost for ER-EIHA and ER-EICA should be higher than DCC assay.
4. ER-EIHA and ER-EICA provide complementary information to standard biochemical assays on the tissue studied, but at present only ER-EIHA and ER-EICA kits can be supplied. Until PR-EIHA and PR-EICA kits are commercially available, biochemical assay, like the dual-labeling assay, which allows simultaneous measurement of both receptors in one tube (Grill et al. 1982; Grill et al. 1984), is superior to ER-EIHA and ER-EICA because time is saved and expenses are lower.

6.1.5 Physiology of Steroid Receptors in Normal Tissues

6.1.5.1 Normal Endometrium

Estrogen increases the level of progesterone receptor in the cytoplasm of the endometrial cell. Progesterone, on the other hand, counteracts the effect of estrogen in four ways:

1. Like the antiestrogens, it inhibits the replenishment of estrogen receptor.
2. It shortens the duration of estrogen retention on the nuclear acceptor.
3. It decreases the level of its own receptor.
4. It increases the level of the enzyme that converts estradiol into the less-active metabolite, estrone (Tseng and Gurpide 1974; Hsueh et al. 1976; MacLaughlin and Richardson 1976).

The levels of total estrogen and progesterone receptor in normal endometrium tend to parallel the serum estrogen levels. The level of unoccupied cytosolic estrogen receptor (ERc) begins to fall before the estrogen peak is reached (Pollow et al. 1978), whereas the level of nuclear estrogen receptor (ERn) and the level of cytosolic progesterone receptor (PRc) tend to parallel the serum estrogen levels (Levy et al. 1980b). In general, the level of ERn is considered a measure of the degree of stimulation by estrogen, and the level of PRc is considered the degree of response; then the level of PRc per unit ERn (PRc/ERn) may be taken as a measure of the sensitivity of the tissue to estrogen.

6.1.5.2 Normal Ovary

The granulosa cells of the ovarian follicle are stimulated to proliferate by estrogen, which increases the amount of ER, and sensitized the cells to a further proliferative stimulus provided by FSH (Richards and Midgley 1976; Richards 1979). Androgens are apparently the physiologic stimulus for follicular atresia and may be the promoters of progesterone biosynthesis (Hillier et al. 1977; Hillier et al. 1981).

Sex steroid receptor-like proteins have been described in bovine, rabbit, and rodent ovaries (Scott and Rennie 1971; Richards 1975; Wilcox and Thorburn 1981), and only recently in normal human ovaries (Punnonen et al. 1979; Jacobs et al. 1980; Milwidsky et al. 1980).

In these experiments the entire ovary was assayed, so that the binding cannot be assigned to any specific ovarian compartment. There were great differences in different laboratory reports on the positive rates and levels of ER and PR of the normal ovary. These differences are still controversial.

6.1.5.3 Normal Cervix

All three tissue components of the normal cervix respond to estrogens. Thus the growth of cervical stroma at puberty, during pregnancy, and during oral contraceptive usage, the mid-cycle secretion of mucus by the columnar epithelium of the endocervix, and the growth of squamous epithelium itself that may be seen on the atrophic postmenopausal cervix treated with hormone replacement are all due to estrogens. It is noted that ERc levels were lower in normal cervix than in normal endometrium and there was no difference in ERn levels between the normal cervix and normal endometrium.

Cytosolic ER and PRc have been measured in normal human endometrium, cervix, ovary, and fallopian tube using one-point saturation DCC assay. Samples were obtained from 69 patients with different gynecologic diseases such as uterine leiomyoma, endometrial carcinoma, benign tumor, ovarian malignant tumor, and tuberculous salpingitis. Levels of ERc and PRc and positive rate in the endometrium were compared with the ERc and PRc levels and positive rate in the cervix, ovary, and fallopian tube and the relationship betweeen pre- and postmenopausal period and the positive rate of ER and PR of the above four tissues was analyzed. It was shown that, in the endometrium, ERc levels were 47 ± 7 fM/mg protein and the positive rate was 80% (40/50); PRc levels were 63 ± 12 fM/mg protein and the positive rate was 78% (39/50). In the cervix, ERc levels were 14 ± 3 fM/mg protein and the positive rate was 38% (19/50) PRc levels were 14 ± 3 fM/mg protein and the positive rate was 40% (20/50). In the ovary, ERc levels were 9 ± 2 fM/mg protein and the positive rate was 30% (15/50); PRc levels were 18 ± 3 fM/mg protein and the positive rate was 48% (24/50). In the fallopian tube, ERc levels were 13 ± 2 fM/mg protein and the positive rate was 44% (22/50); PRc levels were 22 ± 4 fM/mg protein and the positive rate was 60% (30/50). ERc and PRc levels and positive rate were the highest in the endometrium. ERc levels were lower than PRc levels in the ovary. There was no difference between the ERc levels, PRc levels and PRc-positive rates of the endometrium, cervix, and fallopian tube. PR-positive rate in the endometrium was higher in the premenopausal period than the postmenopausal (Wang et al. 1987b).

6.1.6 Estrogen Receptors and Progesterone Receptors in Endometrial Carcinoma

Cytosolic estrogen receptor was present in 75% of cases reported in ten studies (range, 46%–100%) (Grilli et al. 1977; Friberg et al. 1978; Garcia and Rochefort 1979; Martin et al. 1979; McCarty et al. 1979; Soutter et al. 1979; Spona et al. 1979; Young and Ehrlich 1979; Hunter et al. 1980; Ehrlich et al. 1981). There was a tendency for ERc to present more itself frequently in well-differentiated than in poorly differentiated tumors. Almost 80% of ERc-positive cases are also PRc positive. The overall incidence of PRc is 62% of the cases reported in ten studies, ranging from 33% to 89% (MacLaughlin and Richardson 1976; Grilli et al. 1977; Martin et al. 1979; McCarty et al. 1979; Prodi et al. 1979; Spona et al. 1979; Young and Ehrlich 1979; Hunter et al. 1980; Ehrlich et al. 1981).

The relationship to tumor grade is clearer for PRc than ERc, and one-third of the small number of undifferentiated tumors are PRc positive. Nuclear estrogen receptors (ERn) were evaluated in three reports: three of three, seven of eight, and four of four cancers were positive. In 12 of the 15 cases, ERc was also measured as positive (Soutter et al. 1979; Fleming and Gurpide 1980; Geier et al. 1980). Feil et al. (1979) reported that nuclear progesterone receptor (PRn) was positive in 11 of 11 well-differentiated tumors, 11 of 15 moderately differentiated tumors, and 0 of 3 undifferentiated tumors. The PRn of cancers may be different from that of normal tissue since it dissociates more rapidly and is more labile.

The level of ERc and PRc has been found to be proportional to the degree of differentiation of the tumor. A better correlation is obtained with PRc than ERc (McCarty et al. 1979; Hunter et al. 1980; Ehrlich et al. 1981).

Receptor levels do not correlate with the extent of the tumor, e.g., myometrial invasion and extrauterine disease, but the behavior of receptor-positive tumors seems to be less aggressive (Creasman et al. 1980; Hunter et al. 1980). McCarty et al. (1979) reported that only one out of ten patients under the age of 55 years had

ERc or PRc levels below 10 fmol/mg cytosol protein, whereas almost half of the older patients had these low levels. The estrogen production rate in postmenopausal women is related to body weight, but neither weight nor number of years beyond the menopause have been correlated with PRc (Rodriquez et al. 1979). Relatively few patients with endometrial carcinoma are premenopausal and, therefore, the correlation among serum estrogen and progesterone concentration and receptor levels in premenopausal patients is not detectable in this group.

More recently, progestogen treatment has been popular for both recurrent and advanced endometrial carcinoma but the response rate is only about 30% (Smith et al. 1966; Malkasian et al. 1971; Geisler 1973; Reifenstein 1974; Kohorn 1976). The relationship between ERc and PRc levels and clinical response to progestin therapy has been studied (Martin et al. 1979; McCarty et al. 1979; Benraad et al. 1980; Ehrlich et al. 1981). ERc and PRc positivity seems clearly related to a favorable response to progestogen treatment and PRc seems to be a more sensitive predictor than ERc. Li et al. (1989) reported the relationship between ERc and PRc levels and a clinical response to 17β-hydroxyprogesterone caproate in 26 patients with endometrial carcinoma. Seventeen of the 19 ERc- and/or PRc-positive patients (89.5%) responded to 17β-HPC; 1 of the 7 ERc- and PRc-negative patients (14.3%) responded to 17β-HPC. These data suggested that ERc and PRc might be the predictors of progestogen therapy. In the case of ER-positive and PR-positive endometrial carcinoma, progestogen administration should be carried out and in the case of ER-negative and PR-negative endometrial carcinoma, chemotherapy could be used.

6.1.7 Estrogen Receptors and Progesterone Receptors in Ovarian Carcinoma and Cervical Carcinoma

6.1.7.1 Estrogen Receptors and Progesterone Receptors in Ovarian Carcinoma

The common epithelial carcinoma of the ovary is derived from the celomic epithelium, which should be differentiated into müllerian-like tissue. For this reason, it might be expected that these tumors should contain steroid hormone receptors. Since Kiang and Kennedy reported ERc in the ovarian tissue in 1977, a series of studies have been published. These results are shown in Table 6.1.

Kiang and Kennedy (1977) reported the presence of ERc in two of five patients but did not give pathologic or clinical details. Friberg et al. (1978) reported that ERc was found in two out of eight ovarian tumors, a cystadenofibroma in a 73-year-old woman, and a papillary ovarian cancer in a 74-year-old woman. Dihydrotestosterone receptors were found in four of eight tumors, three "mucinous cystadenomas," stages IA, IIB, and IIC in patients aged 22, 32, and 60 years and papillary cancer in a 62-year-old woman. Holt et al. in 1979 reported 16 cases, 8 of which contained ERc, while 3 of the 8 also contained PRc. One of three cases was a grade I–II adenocarcinoma, while the other two were papillary cystadenocarcinomas with metastases. ERc was found in the metastases of two of

Table 6.1. Frequency of cytosolic estrogen receptor (ERc), cytosolic progesterone receptor (PRc), and nuclear estrogen receptor (ERn) in common epithelial cancers of the ovary

Series	Year	ERC (n)	(%)	PRc (n)	(%)	Both (n)	(%)	ERn (n)	(%)
Kiang and Kennedy	1977	2/5	40						
Friberg et al.	1978	2/8	25						
Holt et al.	1979	8/16	50	8/16	50	3/16	19		
Janne et al.	1980	15/21	71	8/21	38	8/21	38		
Holt et al.	1981	15/17	88					12/14	86
Holt et al[a]	1981	9/12	75					3/9	33
Galli et al.	1981	7/10	70	6/10	60	6/10	60		
Hamilton et al.	1981	5/12	42						
Bergqvist et al.	1981	8/11	73	3/8	38	3/8	38		
Hahnel et al.	1982	10/23	43	3/16	19	3/23	19		
Ford et al.	1983	15/39	38	6/39	15	10/49	20		
Willcocks et al.	1983	28/49	57	14/49	29				
Total		124/223	56	48/159	30	33/127	26	15/23	65

[a] Recurrent and metastatic tumors.

the six patients with ERc-positive tumors and metastases available for testing. In the eight patients with recurrent disease, ERc was found in the metastases of four, one to the lung, one to the omentum, and two to the bowel. No receptor was found in three colon and four gastric cancer metastases to the ovary, and none was found in seven of the eight benign ovarian tumors. Janne et al. (1980), who compared 21 malignant tumors, i.e., 6 serous, 1 mucinous, 6 endometrioid, and 8 undifferentiated, with 29 benign tumors, i.e., 8 serous, 18 mucinous, 1 Brenner's and 2 fibromas, and 28 tumor-like lesions, i.e., 13 endometriomas, 13 functional cysts, and 2 polycystic ovaries, found ERc and PRc were present at higher levels in the malignant tumors than in the benign lesions. With the exception of high levels of PRc in endometriosis and luteal cysts, the frequency and levels of receptors were the lowest of all in the tumor-like lesions. Holt et al. (1981) measured the steroid receptor levels by utilizing a single-point saturation assay. The ERc level was higher in this study than those in other studies of primary and recurrent or metastatic ovarian lesions. The study included 30 control tissues, of which all but two, a thecoma and a granulosa cell tumor, were receptor negative. The list of control tissues consisted of 11 dermoids, three thecomas, four granulosa cell tumors, one struma ovarii, and 11 "gut carcinomas" metastasized to the ovary. ERn was measured with a single-point saturation assay after absorption to HPA and was found in 86% of the primary tumors, 33% of their metastases, and all five benign cystadenomas. The study by Galli et al. (1981) included 10 epithelial tumors and 13 disease-free ovaries from women of varying ages. ERc and PRc were measured together with receptors of androgens (ARc) and glucocorticoids (GRc). The receptor levels are low, if there is any in the cancers, but the normal ovaries show a high frequency of binding across the board, ERc accounting for 46%, PRc 54%, ARc 85%, and GRc 92%. Hamilton et al. (1981) found ERc in 5/12 ovarian carcinomas including 4/6 papillary or serous, and 1/1 borderline carcinoma, and ARc in 8/8 including 5 papillary or serous, 1 mucinous, 1 endometrioid, and 1 borderline carcinoma. Bergqvist et al. (1981) included grading as well as histology in their report; both ERc and PRc were present in a GIII serous cystocarcinoma, a GIII serous papillary adenocarcinoma, and a GI mucinous cystadenocarcinoma. No clear relationship among ERc, PRc, grading, and histology was found. The report by Hahnel et al. (1982) included menopausal status, staging, and grading as well as histology. ERc was present in five out of ten serous, one out of four mucinous, and three out of six endometrioid carcinomas, and two out of eight serous (GIII and IV) and one out of four endometrioid (GII) tumors. Of the ERc-positive tumors, three were GII, four were GIII, and three were GIV cancers. Ford et al. (1983), who compared 39 malignant tumors, i.e., 20 serous, 1 endometrioid, and 11 mucinous tumors, with 15 benign tumors, i.e., 7 serous, 7 mucinous, and 1 fibroma tumor, found that four out of eight ERc-positive endometrioid cancers contained PRc as well. In the ten well-differentiated adenocarcinomas, ERc and PRc were found in five and two cases respectively. No ER was found in the 11 mucinous cancers, nor was PR found in the three poorly differentiated adenocarcinomas. ERc and PRc were found in only 1 serous tumor out of 15 benign tumors. The report by Willcocks et al. (1983) on normal ovary, benign ovarian tumor, and malignant tumor is shown in Table 6.2.

6.1.7.2 Estrogen Receptors and Progesterone Receptors in Cervical Cancer

Very few reports have been published on estrogen receptors in cervical tissues. Terenius et al. (1971) measured estradiol binding in 26 cervical carcinomas with a tissue slice method and found very low levels of estrogen receptors in 16 cases. Sanborn et al. (1975) studied the estrogen receptor in the normal cervix tissues

Table 6.2. Distribution of receptors of estrogen (ER) and progesterone (PR) in ovarian tissues. (Adapted from Willcocks et al. 1983)

Receptor status	Normal ovary (n)	(%)	Benign tumors (n)	(%)	Malignant tumors (n)	(%)
ER+/PR+	6	18.8	1	4.0	10	20.4
ER+/PR−	1	3.1	4	16.0	18	36.7
ER−/PR+	18	56.3	3	12.0	4	8.2
ER−/PR−	7	21.9	17	68.0	17	34.7
Total	32		25		49	

and found that estradiol binding was five to ten times lower in the cervical tissue than in the corresponding endometrial tissues. In the report by Syrjala et al. (1978), ERc was found in all three cases of cervical cancer. Hahnel et al. (1979) reported that the proportion of estrogen-receptor-positive tumors was greater in the adenocarcinoma of the cervix (3 of 4) than in the squamous carcinoma of the cervix (7 of 42).

Soutter et al. (1981) reported the distribution of ERc and ERn in squamous cancer of the cervix. Samples of squamous carcinoma contained both ERc and ERn in only 20.9% (9 of 43), ERc alone in 55.8% (24 of 43), ERn alone in 4.7% (2 of 43), and neither ERc nor ERn in 18.6% (8 of 43). Gao et al. (1983) studied the presence or absence of ERc and PRc with a saturation-point dextran-coated charcoal assay in 39 cases of primary cervical carcinoma. The levels of ERc and PRc were compared with clinical stage, histologic type, histologic grade, menstrual status, age, and survival. Both ERc and PRc levels were higher in early-stage cancer, well-differentiated cancer, and adenocarcinoma than in late-stage cancer, poorly differentiated cancer, and squamous carcinoma. A statistically significant difference was found in survival in the PRc($+$) group versus the PRc($-$) group, in the total group, and in the premenopausal patients.

Wang et al. (1987a) reported the incidence and levels of ERc and PRc in 50 squamous cancers of the cervix and 50 noncancerous tissues of the cervix. They compared the incidence of ERc and PRc with staging and menopausal status. ERc levels in the noncancerous tissues were 14 ± 3 fmol/mg protein, PRc levels were 14 ± 3 fmol/mg protein, and ERc($+$) and/or PRc($+$) was found in 9/50 cases (18%). ERc levels in the cancer tissues were 12 ± 3 fmol/mg protein, PRc levels were 9 ± 2 fmol/mg protein, and ERc($+$) and/or PRc($+$) was found in 8/50 cases (16%). Of the 50 squamous cancers of the cervix, 25 were stage II, and 23 were stage III. No significant difference in ERc and PRc levels was found between stage II and stage III ($P > 0.05$) and between premenopausal patients and post-menopausal patients ($P > 0.05$). So far, steroid receptor (SR) determination methods have had the following problems: (a) specificity of binding sites (high-affinity/low-affinity binding sites) and that of the antigenic sites (antibody specificity); (b) receptor accessibility (free/bound receptor, hidden antigenic sites), (c) heterogeneous distribution of receptor tissues.

The importance of SR measurement in making therapeutic decisions is widely accepted for breast cancer and for other target tissues. Studies aiming at correlating the presence of ER and PR in human endometrial carcinoma tissue with response to endocrine therapy have remained controversial. Why did receptors not work so well as predictors of response to endocrine therapy in endometrial carcinoma? One additional explanation could lie in the presence, in the neoplastic cell phenotype, of defects in the steroid receptor pathway, distal to the initial binding of steroid to the receptor. Therefore, it would appear more reliable to look at the end products of hormone action in the form of steroid-induced proteins. The rationale for this would be that by measuring the end products of hormone action instead of receptors one would have a guarantee that all other events preceding hormone binding are working normally.

6.2 Monoclonal Antibody in Cancer

The past 10 years have witnessed the development of tumor immunology. The development of a technique for the production of monoclonal antibodies was an integral part of this revolution.

By combining the nuclei of normal antibody-forming cells with those of their malignant counterparts, Kohler and Milstein (1975) developed an unprecedentedly powerful way of analyzing and purifying individual molecules within the enormously complex mixtures encountered in biologic material. The birth of monoclonal antibody paved the way for subsequent development in tumor immunology.

6.2.1 Basic Principles

6.2.1.1 Immune Response

In mammals, there is a complete immune response. This immune system may serve the perfect immune response and consists of primary lymphoid organs such as marrow, thymus in the adult, secondary lymphoid organs such as lymph nodes, the white pulp of the spleen and mucosa-associated lymphoid tissue (MALT), and other immunologic cells and molecules participating in the immune response. The cardinal features of the immune response might be specificity, memory, amplification, and self-discrimination. The immune response can detect remarkably small chemical differences between foreign materials, e.g., subtly differing strains of influenza virus, minor substitutions of a benzene ring, and the difference between dextro and levo isomers. The memory that develops for previous experience of foreign material may last for the entire life span of the individual. Amplification is the ability of an organism to respond more rapidly and to a greater degree when confronted with the same antigen on a second occassion.

The two important biologic events of immune response – recognition and defense – are to protect the host against a variety of pathogenic materials. Therefore, the stability of inner environment in the host can be maintained. However, it is almost notorious for its capacity to cause inflammatory damage to the host tissues during the course of immune response. This forms the basis of immunopathology such as allergy or hypersensitivity, autoimmunity, lymphoproliferative disease, and immunodeficiency.

Mammalian organisms exhibit cell-mediated and humoral immune response. The characteristics of humoral immune response may be that, when stimulated by appropriately presented antigen, B-lymphocytes transform into activated blast cells which divide to form mature plasma cells secreting immunoglobulin into the extracellular fluids of the body. Immunoglobulins are capable of responding to corresponding antigens and promoting the rejection of these antigens from the host.

6.2.1.2 Polyclonal Antibody and Monoclonal Antibody

Plasma cells proliferated from a B-lymphocyte are called a clone. It has been estimated that approximately 10^8 B cells are formed every day in the bone marrow of a mouse and many more in the bone marrow of a human. This is more than enough to generate the estimated 10^6–10^8 different clones of B cells, each producing a kind of antibody. Some antisera for clinical and laboratory use which were originated from thousands of clones of plasma cells are called polyclonal antibody, which is a mixture of monoclonal antibodies and has heterogeneity. The monoclonal antibody secreted from one clone of plasma cells is a homogeneous antibody.

6.2.1.3 Comparison Between Polyclonal Antibody and Monoclonal Antibody

6.2.1.3.1 Disadvantages of Polyclonal Antibody

Comparative Impurity
Even antibodies of one immunoglobulin class directed against a particular antigenic group do not all have identical combine regions. A variety of different kinds of combining regions can bind one particular antigenic group.

Variability
Variation may be produced among the same species of animal even in different batches of antisera from the same individual animal. The affinity and specificity may be different.

Limited Amount of Antisera
Only a limited amount of antisera could be produced from rabbits, guinea pigs, and sheep.

6.2.1.3.2 Advantages of Monoclonal Antibody

High Specificity
Because they are monospecific and bind to only one determinant per molecule, hybridoma-derived antibodies can be used for the estimation of degree of structural homology between antigens.

Unlimited Amount of Antibody
The production of hybridoma-derived antibody is highly reproducible. If a hybrid cell using a nonsynthesizing plasmacytoma line is prepared, then the hybridoma line will produce only one type of antibody. Thus, whenever a new batch of antibodies is produced from the same cell line, it will have the same specificity.

Producing Monospecific Antibody with Impure Antigen
Fusion can be formed with cells from mice immunized with relatively impure antigen. The need for antigen purification is circumvented by the selection of appropriate cell lines from cloned populations. This, as well as the mono-specificity of the antibody thus obtained, has greatly enhanced the range and sensitivity of potential immunoassay techniques.

Preparing High Specific Labeled Antibody

6.2.2 Procedures for Generating Monoclonal Antibodies

The production of monoclonal antibodies by somatic cell hybridization of antibody-forming cells and continuously replicating cell lines has created a revolution in immunology.

In 1975, Kohler and Milstein fused a mouse myeloma cell line with lymphocytes from a mouse immunized with sheep red blood cells (SRBCs), then the hybrid cells grew continuously in culture, each producing an antibody whose specificity was determined by the genome of the parental lymphocyte. All hybridoma cells were selected using a medium that gradually eliminated the parental myeloma cells, while permitting the hybrids to proliferate. The various hybridomas then were screened for the production of anti-SRBC antibodies. The positive lines then can be cloned, reassayed for antibody production, and then grown in quantity. The technique of hybridoma formation has allowed immunologists to prepare virtually unlimited quantities of antibodies that are chemically, physically, and immunologically completely homogeneous. These molecules are then generally unencumbered by nonspecificity and cross-reactivity.

Having selected suitable plasmacytoma cells, monoclonal antibodies should be prepared through the following steps: immunization, fusion, selection, cloning, and identification (Fig. 6.6).

6.2.3 Application of Monoclonal Antibodies

Although in general the use of monoclonal antibody is still at the research stage, several interesting developments have been reported. Of particular interest is the use of monoclonal antibodies for the definition of cell surface markers for the investigation of specialized or abnormal cell function. This should yield new information on the development and control of the immune system, and perhaps also on the progress of tumorigenesis. Monoclonal antibodies produced by mouse fusion hybrids have many immediate applications in the clinical laboratory as diagnostic or immunoassay reagents.

Monoclonal antibodies might have a therapeutic application in clinical medicine once a suitable human plasmacytoma parent line has been discovered.

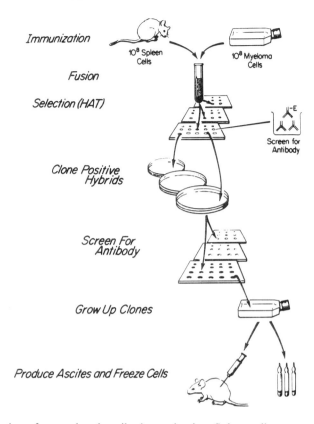

Immunization

Fusion

Selection (HAT)

Clone Positive
Hybrids

Screen For
Antibody

Grow Up Clones

Produce Ascites and Freeze Cells

Fig. 6.6. Schematic illustration of monoclonal antibody production. Spleen cells, sensitized either by in vivo or in vitro immunization, are fused with myeloma cells. The resulting hybridomas are selected by culturing in HAT medium and then screened for production of the desired antibody. Positive cell lines are cloned in soft agar and reassayed for continued antibody production. These antibody-producing hybridomas are grown in quantity by culture or as ascites tumors and then frozen and stored for future use

6.2.3.1 Application of Monoclonal Antibodies in Research on Endocrinology

6.2.3.1.1 Improvement of Hormone Assay

Radioimmunoassays (RIAs) have proliferated and are widely available for measurement of a diverse array of compounds of biologic interest. This technique is based on the competition of radioactively labeled and unlabeled molecules for occupancy of specific binding sites on antibody molecules. The basis for the method is the availability of suitable antibody. Since no two antibody preparations of presumably the same specificity are identical in the distribution of binding constants with an antigenic site, the true concentrations of antibody in a sample cannot be assayed accurately in comparison with a standard antibody preparation, particularly in a range of extremely low concentrations as in RIA, where the equilibrium between the antigen and antibody plays a major role. No standard antibody has become the obstacle in RIA. An unlimited amount of monoclonal antibody can be supplied with the hybridoma technique. Therefore, the standardization would be improved in RIA.

Another type of assay utilizes labeled antibodies. It has been used much less than RIA but it appears to have the potential for wider application. It may be called immunoradiometric assay (IRA). This method differs from RIA in that the antigen to be measured is assayed directly by combination with labeled specific antibodies rather than in competition with a labeled antigen for a limited amount of antibody. In this assay, samples of antigen are reacted with an excess of labeled antibody, and the amount of labeled antibody bound to antigen is determined after removing the unreacted portion of labeled antibody by adsorption on excess immunoadsorbent containing antigen. A reference curve is prepared by the addition of a standard antigen in increasing amounts to a fixed amount of the labeled antibody. The concentration of antigen in test samples is read from observed amounts of bound antibody in the reference curve. This method obviously requires labeled antibody of a high purity and the preparation of an appropriate immunoadsorbent-containing antigen. However, the same immunoadsorbent may be utilized for the preparation of antibody of a high purity prior to or after the labeling. Indeed, the antibodies may be labeled with radioiodine while they are fixed on antigen covalently bound to cellulose and then eluted with acid buffer. Such specifically purified, labeled antibodies may be used successfully in subsequent IRA, which is presently under active investigation for technologic progress as well as for the expansion of application.

6.2.3.1.2. Application of Antibodies in Steroid Receptor Studies

Steroid receptors have classically been studied using hormone-receptor binding activity for their identification and quantitation. Radiolabeled ligands allow highly specific and functional identification of the receptor protein. However, binding ability is labile under certain experimental conditions. Furthermore, in some instances the steroid-binding site is occupied by non-radiolabeled hormones of endogenous or pharmacologic origin. In order to circumvent this problem, monoclonal antibodies offer an alternative method of receptor recognition and quantification, independent of the occupation of the steroid-binding site. The independent recognition of different epitopes on the human estrogen receptor molecule by monoclonal antibodies forms the basis of a new receptor assay (Greene and Jensen 1982).

Monoclonal antibodies to steroid receptors were obtained for the first time by Jensen and coworkers, who immunized rats with estrogen receptor protein purified from the calf uterus (Greene et al. 1980a, b). Hybrioma cell lines, produced by hybridization of Lewis rat spleen cells with a mouse mutant myeloma cell line, secreted antiestrogen receptor immunoglobulins of the M and

G_{2A} classes. None of these clones showed cross-reactivity with receptors from species other than calf. The great majority of antibodies to steroid receptors so far obtained do not have an effect on the interaction of the steroid hormone with its receptor protein.

The DNA-binding domain of the glucocorticoid receptor does not appear to be affected by monoclonal antibodies as assessed by receptor binding to DNA cellulose. There is also evidence in the case of estrogen receptor that monoclonal antibodies (Moncharmont et al. 1982) do not affect the site of interaction with the nuclear component, nor do they interfere with nuclear translocation in vitro (Moncharmont et al. 1982). Furthermore, radiolabeled monoclonal antibodies are able to bind in a specific way to the estrogen receptor in the intact nuclei, when the receptor is already complexed with the acceptor structures (Moncharmont and Parikh 1983). Monoclonal antibodies, by virtue of their specificity for only one antigenic determinant, may be used as an anatomic knife to investigate the subunit structure of a receptor protein. They form stoichiometric complexes with their antigens and, therefore, can provide information on the number of antigenic determinants present on the receptor molecule. Various molecular forms of the calf uterus estrogen receptor have been investigated (Moncharmont et al. 1982; Moncharmont and Parikh 1983). The native "8S" estrogen receptor has been found to have two antigenic determinants per molecule, whereas the "high-salt" 4S form contains only one. This suggests the presence of a homo-dimer of the 4S subunit, associated with yet another protein, in the large "8S" form of the native receptor. The nuclear receptor, which was postulated to be a homodimer of the 4S subunit (Nielsen and Notides 1975; Notides et al. 1975, 1981), has been demonstrated to have two antigenic determinants for the monoclonal antibody tested (Moncharmont et al. 1984).

6.2.3.2 Application of Monoclonal Antibody in the Diagnosis and Therapy of Neoplasms

6.2.3.2.1 Immunodiagnosis of Neoplasms

Gynecologists have long sought a breakthrough in the laboratory diagnosis of cancer, enabling much smaller isolated clones of tumor cells to be detected and the course of cancer to be monitored.

Production of monoclonal immunoglobulins using somatic cell hybridization has stimulated interest in the development of antibodies which recognize tumor-specific or tumor-related antigens and which could be used for immunodiagnosis and immunotherapy (Kohler and Milstein 1975; Diamond et al. 1981). Mono-clonal antibodies have been prepared which are rather selective for several tumors from human, including adenocarcinoma of the colon (Herlyn et al. 1979), neuroblastoma (Kennett et al. 1980), melanoma (Yeh et al. 1979), and carcinoma of the ovary (Bast et al. 1981). The therapeutic and diagnostic applications of these antibodies will depend on their specificity, which must be defined by reactivity with malignant and nonmalignant tissue taken directly from patients as well as with cells in culture.

As described by Bast et al. in 1981, BALB/c mice were immunized with epithelial cell line $OVCA_{433}$ established from ascites fluid from a patient with papillary serous cystadenocarcinoma of the ovary. A clone (OC 125) was selected by screening and flow cytometry using an ovarian cell line, an autologous B-cell line, and cells from a normal ovary. Clones with appropriate specificity were injected intraperitoneally into mice primed with pristane. Antibody was obtained as ascites from hybridoma-bearing animals (Bast et al. 1981). OC 125 can recognize an antigenic determinant (CA 125) which was demonstrated in the derivatives of the celomic epithelium, i.e., the müllerian epithelium in adults. The antigen was also demonstrated in the epithelial cells of the adult fallopian tube, endometrium, and endocervix. OC 125 can detect a normal müllerian-related differentiation antigen which is expressed in certain neoplastic ovarian epithelial cells but not in detectable amounts in normal adult ovarian cells (Kabawat et al. 1983a; Kabawat et al. 1983b).

The discovery of a tumor-specific marker for ovarian cancer might be useful in the early diagnosis of ovarian cancer by means of a simple blood test. An immunoradiometric assay has now been developed to detect CA 125 in the serum from patients with epithelial ovarian carcinomas. ^{125}I-labeled OC 125 may then be used as a probe to detect free CA 125 determinants on the molecules bound to the solid phase in a double determinant "Sandwich" assay (Bast et al. 1983; Klug et al. 1984). Klug et al. reported that serum CA 125 values were 11.2 $\pm$ 5.4 U/ml for 56 apparently healthy adults; serum CA 125 values reached 891 $\pm$ 1544 U/ml for 105 patients with ovarian carcinoma; and these values were 10–100 times higher than that for apparently healthy adults (Klug et al. 1984). In one study reported by Bast et al., serum CA 125 values were more than 35 U/ml in 0.1% (1/888 cases) of apparently healthy individuals; in 4% (6/143 cases) of patients with nonmalignant diseases; and in 82% (83/101 cases) of patients with ovarian carcinoma. In this report, serum specimens were obtained from 38 patients on 2–18 occassions over 2–60 months. A doubling or halving of antigen levels is considered a significant change, and CA 125 antigen levels correlated with clinical course in 42 of 45 instances (93%). The rising CA 125 levels were associated with disease progression in all of the 17 cases.

In one patient with stage IV poorly differentiated endometrioid ovarian carcinoma, it was possible to monitor CA 125 levels on ten occasions over 60 months. After surgical cytoreduction and chemotherapy, CA 125 levels decreased from 7828 to 86 U/ml. With additional treatment, CA 125 levels fell to normal. "Second-look" laparoscopies failed to reveal residual tumor, and further treatment was discontinued pending disease progression. When the patient had no symptoms that could be attributed to tumor growth, an increase in CA 125 was observed. This increase in CA 125 appeared 7 months before the earliest evidence of disease recurrence was obtained by noninvasive techniques. With the progressed disease, CA 125 levels increased gradually and rose to 2514 U/ml before her death. CA 125 promises to provide a clinically useful marker for monitoring the response to treatment in the majority of patients with epithelial ovarian cancer (Bast et al. 1983).

Niloff et al. reported that, among 29 patients with endometrial carcinoma, CA 125 levels increased in 14 of the 18 patients (77.8%) who had stage IV or recurrent disease but in none of the 11 patients who had stage I and stage II tumors at presentation (Niloff et al. 1984). In a report presented by the Cancer Institute Hospital, Beijing, elevated levels of CA 125 (35 U/ml) were found in sera from each of the 6 patients with stage IV or uncontrolled endometrial carcinoma; from 2 of the 5 patients with stage III endometrial carcinoma; and from 8 of the 34 patients with stage I or II endometrial carcinoma (Table 6.3) (Wu et al. 1988).

Among the patients with endometrial carcinoma, CA 125 levels were elevated in those who had advanced or recurrent disease but not in those who had early-stage tumors confined to the uterus. Possibly, a substantial quantity of tumor must be present to produce enough antigen to cause an elevation in the serum. Alternatively, antigen shed into the uterine cavity may not find its way into the peripheral circulation.

6.2.3.2.2. Monoclonal Antibody Therapy of Cancer

The objective of cancer chemotherapy is to destroy malignant cells while minimizing damage to normal cells and tissues. But at present the differential cytotoxicity of chemotherapeutic agents between tumor cells and normal cells is not sufficient to permit curative doses to be administered without producing unacceptable toxic manifestations. Monoclonal antibodies that recognize human tumors offer new approaches to targeting antitumor agents. It is hoped that "magic bullets" for cancer therapy can be achieved by using monoclonal antibodies, either given alone or used as carriers of antitumor agents. Antibody targeting of drugs to tumors requires that the antibody localizes in the tumor and also uniformly penetrates regions of the tumor that contribute to its progressive growth. Also the antibody should not react with the normal tissues or at least

Table 6.3. Detection of CA 125 antigen in serum of patients with endometrial carcinoma

Stage	Patients (n)	>35 u/ml (n)	(%)	>65 u/ml (n)	%
I	21	5	23.8	3	14.2
II	13	3	23.0	3	23.0
III	5	2	40.0	2	40.0
IV	5	5	100.0	5	100.0
Uncontrolled	1	1	100.0	1	100.0
Total	45	16	35.5	14	31.1

this reactivity should be sufficiently low so as to permit preferential uptake into the tumor tissue. Conjugation of drugs to antibody molecules aims to introduce the maximum number of residues using conditions that ensure optimal retention of both drug and antibody reactivities. Antibody conjugates have been synthesized with a number of anticancer agents including chlorambucil, P-phenylenediamine mustard, daunomycin, Adriamycin, methotrexate, vindesine, and cytosine 1-β-D-arahinofuranoside.

Drug-antibody conjugates have been shown to inhibit growth of human tumor xenografts (Baldwin et al. 1985) and have clearly demonstrated a marked reduction in toxicity (Baldwin et al. 1986). The selection of monoclonal antibodies that can be used for drug targeting will depend on related investigations showing that they do localize in human tumors. In this respect, a number of factors will have to be taken into consideration.

First, antigen modulation following monoclonal antibody interaction with tumor cells is a potentially limiting factor in drug-antibody targeting. Second, it is now quite clear that there is often a marked variation of antigen expression in human tumors. Third, the generation of antibodies in patients to injected murine monoclonal antibody or the attached drug moiety that will function as a haptenic group must be recognized as a potentially limiting factor.

Monoclonal antibodies linked to protein toxins (immunotoxins) are a new class of pharmacologic reagents. They combine the exquisite cell-type selectivity of monoclonal antibodies with the potent toxicity of ricin and diphtheria toxin. Two types of immunotoxins have been made, each with different advantages. In vivo trials of immunotoxins in animal models of cancer therapy have shown small but reproducible therapeutic efficacy. Limitations appear to be slow kinetics of ricin A chain immunotoxins, rapid clearance or inactivation of immunotoxins in vivo, and a diffusion barrier for access of intravenous immunotoxins to extravascular tumor cells.

One important research area that will further the use of immunotoxins is the study of how toxins and toxin conjugates enter the cytosol of cells. Another promising direction is the use of genetic engineering to custom design new toxins for chemotherapy. It is hoped that imaginative new designs at the gene levels will allow us to increase the target cell toxicity of immunotoxins and decrease the side effects to the recipient.

The use of monoclonal antibodies and antibody immunoconjugates in the treatment of cancer is in its infancy. Problems such as nonspecific localization of antibody in the reticuloendothelial system, host antibody response, and antigenic heterogenecity are all major obstacles to safe and effective treatment with monoclonal antibodies. These issues have been under investigation in animal models and humans. Perhaps the most important future role of monoclonal antibody therapy will be in the patients with minimal disease in the adjuvant setting, in whom antibody conjugates may localize and destroy micrometastatic deposits of tumor cells. One should remain cautiously optimistic in exploring these exciting new approaches to cancer therapy.

References

Anderson JN, Clark JH, Peck EJ Jr (1972) The relationship between nuclear receptor estrogen binding and uterotrophic responses. Biochem Biophys Res Commun 48:1460–1468

Baldwin RW, Durrant L, Embleton MJ et al. (1985) Design and therapeutic evaluation of monoclonal antibody 791T/36-methotrexate conjugates. UCLA symposium, MoAbs & cancer therapy, Los Angeles, Jan 26–Feb 2, 1985

Baldwin RW, Embleton MJ, Gallego J et al. (1986) Monoclonal antibody drug conjugates for cancer therapy. In: Roth JA (ed) Monoclonal antibody in cancer. Advances in diagnosis and treatment. Futura, New York, 215–257

Barrows GH, Stroupe SB, Richm JD (1980) Nuclear uptake of ethylsuccinamide bridged 17-beta-estradiol-fluorescein as a marker of estrogen receptor activity. Am J Clin Pathol 73:330–339

Bast RC Jr, Feeney M, Lazarus H et al. (1981) Reactivity of a monoclonal antibody with human ovarian carcinoma. J Clin Invest 68:1331–1337

Bast RC Jr, Klug TL, St John E et al. (1983) A radioimmunoassay using a monoclonal antibody to monitor the course of epithelial ovarian cancer. N Engl J Med 309:883–887

Baxter JD, Funder JW (1979) Hormone receptor. N Engl J Med 301:1149–1161

Benraad TJ, Friberg LG, Koenders AJM et al. (1980) Do estrogen and progesterone receptors (E_2R and PR) in metastazing endometrial cancers predict the response to gestogen therapy? Acta Obstet Gynecol Scand 59:155–159

Bergqvist A, Kullander S, Thorell J (1981) A study of estrogen and progesterone cytosol receptor concentration in benign and malignant ovarian tumors and a review of malignant ovarian tumors treated with medroxyprogesterone acetate. Acta Obstet Gynecol Scand [Suppl]101:75–81

Byar DP, Sears ME, McGuire WL (1979) Relationship between estrogen receptor values and clinical data in predicting the response to endocrine therapy for patients with advanced breast cancer. Eur J Cancer 15:299–310

Carlson RA, Gorski J (1980) Characterization of a unique population of unfilled estrogen-binding sites associated with the nuclear fraction of immature rat uterus. Endocrinology 106:1776–1785

Chamness GC, Mercer WD, McGuire WL (1980) Are histochemical methods for estrogen receptor valid? J Histochem Cytochem 28:792–798

Charpin C, Martin PM, Jacquemier J et al. (1986) Estrogen receptor immunocytochemical assay (ER-ICA) computerized image analysis system, immunoelectron microscopy and comparisons with estradiol binding assays in 115 breast carcinomas. Cancer Res 46:4271s–4277s

Consensus Meeting on Steroid Receptors in Breast Cancer, Bethesda, June 1979, p 27–29

Creasman WT, McCarty KS, Barton TK et al. (1980) Clinical correlates of estrogen and progesterone-binding proteins in human endometrial adenocarcinoma. Obstet Gynecol 55:363–370

Dandliker WB, Brauwn RJ, Hsu ML et al. (1978) Investigation for hormone-receptor interactions by means of fluorescence labelling. Cancer Res 38:4212–4224

DeSombre ER, Greene GL, King WT, Jensen EV (1984) Estrogen receptors, antibodies and hormone dependent cancer. In: Gurpide E, Calandra, Levy C, Soto RJ (eds) Hormones and Cancer. Liss, New York, Vol 142, 1–21

DeSombre ER, Thorpe SM, Rose C et al. (1986) Prognostic usefulness of estrogen receptor immunocytochemical assays for human breast cancer. Cancer Res 46:4256s–4264s

Diamond BA, Yelton DE, Sharff MD (1981) Monoclonal antibodies. N Engl J Med 304:1344–1349

Edwards DP, Martin PM, Horwitz KB et al. (1980) Subcellular compartmentalization of estrogen receptors in human breast cancer cells. Exp Cell Res 127:197–213

Ehrlich CE, Young PCM, Cleary RE (1981) Cytoplasmic progesterone and estradiol receptors in normal, hyperplasmic and carcinomatous endometria: therapeutic implications. Am J Obstet Gynecol 141:539–546

Feil P, Maun W Jr, Mortel R, Bardin CW (1979) Nuclear progestin receptors in normal and malignant human endometrium. J Clin Endocrinol Metab 48:327–334

Fleming H, Gurpide E (1980) Available estradiol receptors in nuclei from endometrium. J Steroid Biochem 13:3–11

Ford LC, Berek JS, Lagasse LD et al. (1983) Estrogen and progesterone receptors in ovarian neoplasma. Gynecol Oncol 15:299–304

Friberg LG, Kullander S, Persijn JP, Korsten CB (1978) On receptors for estrogens (E_2) and androgens (DHT) in human endometrial carcinoma and ovarian tumors. Acta Obstet Gynecol Scand 57:265–271

Furmanski P, Saunders DE, Brooks SC, Rich MA (1980) The prognostic value of estrogen receptor determinations in patients with primary breast cancer: an update. Cancer 46:2794–2796

Galli MC, DeGiovanni C, Nicoletti G et al. (1981) The occurrence of multiple steroid hormone receptors in disease-free and neoplastic human ovary. Cancer 47:1297–1302

Gao YL, Twiggs LB, Leung BS et al. (1983) Cytoplasmic estrogen and progesterone receptors in primary cervical carcinoma: clinical and histopathologic correlates. Am J Obstet Gynecol 146:299–306

Garcia M, Rochefort H (1979) Evidence and characterization of the binding of two 3H-labeled androgens to the estrogen receptor. Endocrinology 104:1797–1809

Geier A, Beery R, Levran D et al. (1980) Unoccupied nuclear receptors for estrogen in human endometrial tissue. J Clin Endocrinol Metab 50:541–545

Geisler HE (1973) The use of megestrol acetate in the treatment of advanced malignant lesions of the endometrium. Gynecol Oncol 1:340–344

Greene GL, Jensen EV (1982) Monoclonal antibodies as probes for estrogen receptor detection and characterization. J Steroid Biochem 16:353–359

Greene GL, Fitch FW, Jensen EV (1980a) Monoclonal antibodies to estrophilin: probes for the study of estrogen receptors. Proc Natl Acad Sci USA 77:157–161

Greene GL, Nolan C, Engler JP, Jensen EV (1980b) Monoclonal antibodies to human estrogen receptors. Proc Natl Acad Sci USA 77:5115

Grill HJ, Manz B, Pollow K (1982) Double-labeling assay system for estrogen and progesterone receptors. Lancet 1:679

Grill HJ, Manz B, Belovsky O, Pollow K (1984) Criteria for the establishment of a double-labeling assay for simultaneous determination of estrogen and progesterone receptors. Oncology 41:25–32

Grilli S, Ferreri A, Gola G et al. (1977) Cytoplasmic receptors for 17β-estradiol, 5α-hydroxytestasterone and progesterone in normal and abnormal human uterine tissues. Cancer Lett 2:247–258

Hahnel R, Martin JD, Masters AM et al. (1979) Estrogen receptors and blood hormone levels in cervical carcinoma and other gynecological tumors. Gynecol Oncol 8:226–233

Hahnel R, Kelsall GRH, Martin JD et al. (1982) Estrogen and progesterone receptors in tumors of the human ovary. Gynecol Oncol 13:145–151

Hamilton TC, Daview P, Griffiths K (1981) Androgen and oestrogen binding in cytosols of human ovarian tumors. J Endocrinol 91:421–431

Herlyn M, Steplewshi Z, Herlyn D, Koprowski H (1979) Cororectal carcinoma-specific antigen: detection by means of monoclonal antibodies. Proc Natl Acad Sci USA 76:1438–1442

Hillier SG, Knazek RA, Ross GT (1977) Androgenic stimulation of progesterone production by granulosa cells from preantral follicles: further in vitro studies using replicate cell cultures. Endocrinology 100:1539–1549

Hillier SG, Reichert JE Jr, Van Hall EV (1981) Control of preovulatory follicular estrogen biosynthesis in the human ovary. J Clin Endocrinol Metab 52:847–856

Holt JA, Caputo TA, Kelly KM et al. (1979) Estrogen and progestin binding in cytosols of ovarian adenocarcinoma. Obstet Gynecol 53:50–58

Holt JA, Lyttle CR, Lorincz MA et al. (1981) Estrogen receptor and peroxidase activity in epithelial ovarian carcinoma. JNCI 67:307–318

Horwitz RI, Feinstein AR, Vidone RA et al. (1981) Histopathologic distinctions in the relationship of estrogens and endometrial cancer. JAMA 246:1245–1247

Hsueh AJW, Peck EJ Jr, Clark JH (1976) Control of uterine estrogen receptor levels by progesterone. Endocrinology 98:438–444

Hunter RE, Longcope C, Jordan VC (1980) Steroid hormone receptors in adenocarcinoma of the endometrium. Gynecol Oncol 10:152–161

Jacobs BR, Suchocki S, Smith RG (1980) Evidence for a human ovarian progesterone receptor. Am J Obstet Gynecol 138:332–336

Janne O, Kauppila A, Syrjala P, Vihko R (1980) Comparison of cytosol estrogen and progestin receptor status in malignant and benign tumors and tumor-like lesions of human ovary. Int J Cancer 25:175–179

Jensen EV (1962) Basic guides to the mechanism of estrogen action. Recent Prog Horm Res 18:387–414

Jensen EV, Suzuki T, Kawashina T et al. (1968) A two-step mechanism for the interaction of estradiol with rat uterus. Proc Natl Acad Sci USA 59:632–638

Jensen EV, Green GL, Closs LE, DeSombre ER (1979) The immunoendocrinology of estrophilin. Adv Exp Med Biol 117:1–16

Jordan VC, Jacobson HI, Keenan EJ (1986) Determination of estrogen receptor in breast cancer using monoclonal antibody technology: results of a multicenter study in the United States. Cancer Res 46:4237s–4240s

Jungblut PW, Kallweit E, Sierralta W et al. (1978) The occurrence of steroidfree 'activated' estrogen receptor in target cell nuclei. Hoppe-Seyler's Z Physiol Chem 359:1259–1268

Kabawat SE, Bast RC Jr, Welch WR et al. (1983a) Immunopathologic characterization of a monoclonal antibody that recognizes common surface antigens on human ovarian tumors of serous, endometrioid and clear cell types. Am J Clin Pathol 79:98–104

Kabawat SE, Bast RC Jr, Bshn AK et al. (1983b) Tissue distribution of a coelomicepithelium-related antigen recognized by the monoclonal antibody OC 125. Int J Gynecol Pathol 2:275–285

Kennett RH, Jonak ZL, Bechtol KB (1980) Monoclonal antibodies against human tumor-associated antigens. In: Kennet RH et al. (eds) Monoclonal antibodies. Plenum, New York, p 155

Kiang DT, Kennedy BJ (1977) Estrogen receptor assay in the differential diagnosis of adenocarcinoma. JAMA 238:32–34

King RJB (1979) Effects of estrogen and progesterone treatments on endometrial from postmenopausal women. Cancer Res 39(3):1094–1101

King WJ, Greene GL (1984) Monoclonal antibodies localize estrogen receptor in the nuclei of target cells. Nature 307:745–747

King RJB, Raju KS, Siddle NC et al. (1983) Simple biochemical method to assess progestin effects on human endometrial DNA synthesis and its application to endometrial carcinoma. Cancer Res 43:5033–5036

King WJ, DeSombre ER, Jensen EV, Greene GL (1985) Comparison of immunochemical and steroid binding assays for estrogen receptor in human breast tumors. Cancer Res 45:293–304

Klug TL, Bast RC Jr, Niloff JM et al. (1984) A monoclonal antibody immunoradiometric assay for an antigenic determinant (CA-125) associated with human epithelial ovarian carcinoma. Cancer Res 44:1048–1053

Kohler G, Milstein C (1975) Continuous cultures of fused cells, secreting antibody of predefined specificity. Nature 256:495–497

Kohorn EI (1976) Gestagens and endometrial carcinoma. Gynecol Oncol 4:398–411

Kurzon RM, Sternberger LA (1978) Estrogen receptor immunocytochemistry. J Histochem Cytochem 26:803–808

Leclercq G, Bojar H, Goussard J et al. (1986) Abbott monoclonal enzyme immunoassay measurement of estrogen receptors in human breast cancer: a European multicenter study. Cancer Res 46:4233S–4236S

Lee SH (1978) Cytochemical study of estrogen receptor in human mammary cancer. Am J Clin Pathol 70:197–203

Levy C, Mortel R, Eychenne B et al. (1980a) Unoccupied nuclear aestradiol-receptor sites in normal human endometrium. Biochem J 185:733–738

Levy C, Robel P, Gantray JP et al. (1980b) Estradiol and progesterone receptors in human endometrium: normal and abnormal menstrual cycles and early pregnancy. Am J Obstet Gynecol 136:646–651

Li SY, Wang EY, Li JX (1988) Cytosol estrogen, progesterone receptor levels as indexes of response to hormone therapy in endometrial carcinoma. J Pract Oncol 28–32

Liu YX (1981) Estradiol and progesterone receptors assay. Reprod Contraception 1:53–56

Lowry OH, Rosenbrough NJ, Farr AL, Randall RJ (1951) Protein measurement with the folin phenol reagent. J Biol Chem 193:265–275

MacLaughlin DT, Richardson GS (1976) Progesterone binding by normal and abnormal human endometrium. J Clin Endocrinol Metab 42:667–678

Magdelenat H, Merle S, Zajdela A (1986) Enzyme immunoassay of estrogen receptors in fine needle aspirates of breast tumors. Cancer Res 46:4265s–4270s

Malkasian GD, Decker DG, Mussey E, Johnson CG (1971) Progestin treatment of recurrent endometrial carcinoma. Am J Obstet Gynecol 110:15–23

Markaverich BM, Williams M, Upchurch S, Clark JH (1981a) Heterogeneity of nuclear estrogen binding sites in rat uterus: a simple method for the quantitation of type I and type II sites by ^{3}H-estradiol exchange. Endocrinology 109:62–69

Markaverich BM, Upchurch S, McCormack SA et al. (1981b) Differential stimulation of uterine cells by nafoxidine and clomiphene: relationship between nuclear estrogen receptors and type II estrogen binding sites and cellular growth. Biol Reprod 24:171–181

Martin PM, Horwitz KB, Ryan D, McGuire WL (1978a) Phytoestrogen interaction with estrogen receptors in human breast cancer. Endocrinology 103:1860–1867

Martin PM, Rolland PH, Jacquemier J et al. (1978b) Multiple steroid receptors in human breast cancer I. Technological features. Biomedicine 28:278–287

Martin PM, Rolland PH, Gammerre M et al. (1979) Estradiol and progesterone receptors, histopathological examinations and clinical responses under pregestin therapy. Int J Cancer 23:321–329

Martin PM, Sheridan PJ (1982) Towards a new model for the mechanism of action of steroids. J Steroid Biochem 16:215–229

Martin PM, Magdelenat H, Benyahia B et al. (1983) New approach for visualizing estrogen receptors in target cells using inherent fluorescent ligands and image intensification. Cancer Res 43:4956–4965

McCarty KS Jr, Barton TK, Fetter BF et al. (1979) Correlation of estrogen and progesterone receptors with histologic differentiation in endometrial adenocarcinoma. Am J Pathol 96:171–182

McCarty KS Jr., Miller LS, Cox EB et al. (1985) Estrogen receptor and immunohisto-chemical methods using monoclonal antireceptor antibodies. Arch Pathol Lab Med 109:716–721

McCarty KS Jr, Szabo E, Flowers JL et al. (1986) Use of a monoclonal antiestrogen receptor antibody in the immunohistochemical evaluation of human tumors. Cancer Res 46:4244s–4248s

McClelland RA, Bergen U, Miller LS et al. (1986) Immunocytochemical assay for estrogen receptor: relationship to outcome of therapy in patients with advanced breast cancer. Cancer Res 46:4241s–4243s

McGuire WL, Carbone PP, Sears ME, Escher GC (1975) Estrogen receptors in breast cancer: an overview. In: McGuire WL et al. (eds.) Estrogen receptors in human breast cancer. Raven, New York, 1–7

Milwidsky A, Younes MA, Besch NF et al. (1980) Receptor-like binding proteins for testosterone and progesterone in the human ovary. Am J Obstet Gynecol 138:93–98

Moncharmont B, Parikh I (1983) Binding of monoclonal antibodies to the nuclear estrogen receptor in intact nuclei. Biochem Biophys Res Commun 114:107

Moncharmont B, Su JL, Parikh I (1982) Monoclonal antibodies against estrogen receptor: interaction with different molecular forms and functions of the receptor. Biochemistry 21:6916–6921

Moncharmont B, Anderson WL, Rosenberg B, Parikh I (1984) Interaction of estrogen receptor of calf uterus with a monoclonal antibody: probing of various molecular forms. Biochemistry 23:3907–3912

Nenci I, Beccati MD, Piffanelli A, Lanza G (1976) Detection and dynamic localization of estradiol-receptor complexes in intact target cells by immunofluorescence technique. J Steroid Biochem 7:505–510

Nicholson RI, Griffiths K, Colin P et al. (1986) Evaluation of an enzyme immunoassay for estrogen receptors in human breast cancers. Cancer Res 46:4299s

Nielsen S, Notides AC (1975) Transformation of the rat uterine estrogen receptor after partial purification. Biochem Biophys Acta 381:377–383

Niloff JM, Klug TL, Schaetzl E et al. (1984) Elevation of serum CA 125 in carcinomas of the fallopian tube, endometrium and endocervix. Am J Obstet Gynecol 148:1057–1058

Notides AC, Hamilton DE, Auer HE (1975) A kinetic analysis of the estrogen receptor transformation. J Biol Chem 250:3945–3950

Notides AC, Lerner N, Hamilton DE (1981) Positive cooperativity of the estrogen receptor. Proc Natl Acad Sci, USA 78:4926–4930

Noyes AT, Hertig AT, Rock J (1950) Dating the endometrial biopsy. Fertil Steril 1:3–25

O'Malley BW, Schrader WT (1976) The receptors of steroid hormones. Sci Am 234:(2):22–43

Pertschuk LP, Tobin EH, Brigati DJ et al. (1978) Immunofluorescent detection of estrogen receptor in breast cancer: comparison with dextran-coated charcoal and sucrose gradient assays. Cancer 41:907–911

Pollow K, Schmidt-Gollwitzer M, Pollow B (1978) Progesterone- and estradiolbinding proteins from normal human endometrium and endometrial carcinoma: a comparative study. In: Wittliff JI, Dapunt O (eds) Steroid dependent neoplasia. Innsbruck

Press MF, Greene GL (1984) An immunocytochemical method for demonstrating estrogen receptor in human uterus using monoclonal antibodies to human estrophilin. Lab Invest 50:480–486

Press MF, Nousek-Goebl NA, Greene GL (1985) Immunoelectron microscopic localization of estrogen receptor with monoclonal estrophilin antibodies. J Histochem Cytochem 33:915–924

Prodi G, DeGiovanni C, Galli MC et al. (1979) 17β-Estradiol, 5α-dihydrotestosterone, progesterone and cortisol receptors in normal and neoplastic human endometrium. Tumori 65:241–253

Punnonen R, Kouvoven L, Lovgren T, Rouramo L (1979) Uterine and ovarian estrogen receptor levels in climacteric women. Acta Obstet Gynecol Scand 58:389

Reifenstein EC (1974) The treatment of advanced endometrial cancer with hydroxyprogesterone caproate. Gynecol Oncol 2:377–391

Richards JS (1975) Content of nuclear estradiol complex in rat corpora lutea during pregnancy – relationship to estrogen concentration and cytosol receptor availability. Endocrinology 96:227–414

Richards JS (1979) Hormonal control of ovarian follicular development: a 1978 perspective. Recent Prog Horm Res 35:230–343

Richards JS, Midgley AR Jr (1976) Protein hormone action: a key to understanding ovarian and follicular luteal cell development. Biol Reprod 14:82

Robboy SJ, Bradley R (1979) Changing trends and prognostic features in endometrial cancer associated with exogenous estrogen therapy. Obstet Gynecol 54:269

Rodriquez J, Sen KK, Seski JC et al. (1979) Progesterone binding by human endometrial tissue during the proliferative and secretory phase of the menstrual cycle and by hyperplastic and carcinomatous endometrium. Am J Obstet Gynecol 133:660–665

Sanborn BM, Held B, Kuo HS (1975) Specific estrogen binding proteins in human cervix. J Steroid Biochem 6:1107–1112

Scatchard G (1949) The attraction of protein for small molecules and ions. Ann NY Acad Sci 51:660–672

Scott RS, Rennie PIC (1971) An estrogen receptor in the corpus luteum of the pseudopregnant rabbit. Endocrinology 89:297–301

Sheridan PJ, Buchanan JM, Anselmo VC, Martin PM (1980) Equilibrium of the intracellular distribution of steroid receptors. Nature 282:579–582

Singhakowinta A, Saunders DE, Brooks SC et al. (1980) Clinical application of estrogen receptor in breast cancer. Cancer 46:2932–2938

Sirbasku DA, Leland SE, Benson RH (1981) Properties of a growth factor activity present in crude extracts of rat uterus. J Cell Physiol 107:345–358

Smith JP, Rutledge F, Soffar SW (1966) Progestins in the treatment of patients with endometrial adenocarcinoma. Am J Obstet Gynecol 94:977–984

Sonnenschein C, Soto AM (1980a) But ... are estrogens per se growth-promoting hormones? JNCI 64:211–215

Sonnenschein C, Soto AM (1980b) The mechanism of estrogen action: the old and a new paradigm. In: McLachlan JA (ed) Estrogens in the environment. Elsevier, Amsterdam

Soutter WP, Hamilton K, Leake RE (1979) High affinity binding of oestradiol-17β in the nuclei of human endometrial cells. J Steroid Biochem 10:529–534

Soutter WP, Pegoraro RJ, Green-Thompson RW et al. (1981) Nuclear and cytoplasmic oestrogen receptors in squamous carcinoma of the cervix. Br J Cancer 44:154–159

Spona J, Ulm R, Bieglmayer C, Husslein P (1979) Hormone serum levels and hormone receptor contents of endometria in women with normal menstrual cycles and patients bearing endometrial carcinoma. Gynecol Obstet Invest 10:71–80

Syrjala P, Kontula K, Janne O et al. (1978) Steroid receptors in normal and neoplastic human uterine tissue. In: Brush MG et al. (eds) Endometrial cancer. Bailliere Tindall, London, p 242–251

Terenius L, Lindell A, Persson BH (1971) Binding of oestradiol-17 to human cancer tissue of the female genital tract. Cancer Res 31:1895

Thorpe Sm, Lykkesfeldt AE, Vinterby A, Lonsdorfer M (1986) Quantitative immunological detection of estrogen receptors in nuclear pellets from human breast cancer biopsies. Cancer Res 46:4251s–4255s

Tseng L, Gurpide E (1974) Induction of human endometrial estradiol dehydrogenase by progestins. Endocrinology 97:824–833

Wang EY, Li Sy, Liu ZM et al (1987a) Cytosol estrogen, progesterone receptor levels in non-cancerous cervix and squamous cell carcinoma of cervix. Pract J Cancer 2:1–4

Wang EY, Li SY, Liu ZM (1987b) Cytosol estrogen, progesterone receptor levels in non-cancerous cervix, endometrium, ovary and fallopian tube. J Practical Oncol 1:11–13

Welshous WV, Lieberman ME, Gorski J (1984) Nuclear localization of unoccupied oestrogen receptors. Nature 307:747–749

Wilcox DL, Thorburn GD (1981) Progesterone binding protein in the bovine corpus lutem. J Steroid Biochem 14:841–850

Willcocks D, Toppila M, Hudson CN et al. (1983) Estrogen and progesterone receptors in human ovarian tumors. Gynecol Oncol 16:246–253

Wu AR, Wang EY, Li Ling (1989) The application of monoclonal antibody OC 125 in gynecological oncology. J Exp Clin Cancer Res 8:29–37

Yalow RS, Berson SA (1960) Immunoassay of endogenous plasma insulin in man. J Clin Invest 39:1157–1175

Yeh MY, Hellstrom I, Brown JP et al. (1979) Cell surface antigens of human melanoma identified by monoclonal antibody. Proc Natl Acad Sci USA 167:2927–2831

Young PCM, Ehrlich CE (1979) Progesterone receptors in human endometrial cancer. In: Thompson EB, Lippman ME (eds) Steroid receptors and the management of cancer. CPC Press, Boca Raton, 1:135–160

Zava DT, McGuire WL (1977) Estrogen receptor. Unoccupied sites in nuclei of breast tumor cell line. J Biol Chem 252:3703–3708

Zhang HJ, Li SY, Li ZQ, Fei LM (1983) Estrogen receptors activity assay by DEAE (Di-Ethyl-Amino-Ethyl) cellulose paper method. J Chin Oncol 5:110–113

7 Medicopsychologic Problems
in Patients with Gynecologic Cancers

The life process of all persons involves a continuous interchange between the internal and external environments. It is characterized by input-interaction-output phenomena in consistent, often cyclic or repetitive, patterns of behavior. Both mankind and his environment are dynamic energy fields. Unity between them is evidenced by pattern and organization within their reciprocal relationship. Under stressful circumstances, the individual will favor behavioral reactions that have been helpful in crises in the past. There is a specific pattern to the entire process of disorganizations to reorganization through the resolution of the crisis (Aguilera and Messick 1974). Behavior of the human organization when faced with the problem of cancer is an example of the result of a force in the human field that is great enough to alter the speed of change in the life process of the patient.

In spite of wide publicity regarding high cure rates for many types of cancer that are detected and treated early, many people are convinced that, once a diagnosis of cancer has been made, a death warrant has been signed. This traditional and psychologically ingrained concept of cancer and its implications are reflected in the question: "Doctor, do I have cancer?" The manner in which an individual will react to a diagnosis of cancer will depend on her ability to adapt to situations of threat. It will also depend on chronologic age, emotional maturity, established patterns of behavior in relation to stress, family relationships, and what the person believes about cancer. As a result, the individual may employ any one of a variety of techniques in attempts to cope with the situation. It is essential, therefore, that the medical staff understand these various tactics and be able to recognize the approach the individual is using to grapple with these stressful situations. To intelligently and psychologically assist this patient, it is wise to consider the impact of cancer itself, the patterns of adjustment used by the person, and the various beliefs people have concerning the cause of cancer. (Du 1987, Lin 1987).

7.1 Psychologic Problems in Patients with Gynecologic Cancers

7.1.1 Concept of Psychologic Stress

Stress is a special tense condition produced by the person who reacts to the disturbances of stimulus. It represents either the interactive results among the tense stimuli, personal physiologicopsychologic characteristics and environ-

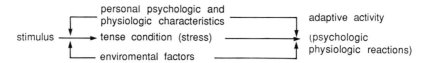

Fig. 7.1. Diagram of stress

mental factors, or the secondary excitant of eventual adaptive activity (psychologic and physiologic reactions) (Fig. 7.1).

Psychologic stress is a part of the whole and may cause a series of psychologic reactions, e.g., anxiety, emotional release, learned helplessness, impairment of cognition, and misconception about self-worth. Cancer itself is a tense stimulus for the patients with gynecologic cancers provoking a series of psychologic reactions.

7.1.2 Psychologic Stress in Each Stage of Medical Course

Two stages and five phases are included in the process of psychologic stress with the development of illness and course of treatment.

7.1.2.1 Pretreatment Stage

The pretreatment stage is the period before being consulted by physicians and includes two phases:

7.1.2.1.1 Phase of Experiencing Symptoms Suffered

7.1.2.1.2 Phase of Being Supposed a Patient

Each of the symptoms caused by the illness and the subjective experience of being an uncertain patient might be sources of psychologic stress for the patient.

7.1.2.2 Treatment Stage

7.1.2.2.1 Phase of Contact with Physicians

The threat presented by the symptoms and the course of being consulted by physicians might be sources of psychologic stress for the patient.

7.1.2.2.2 Phase of Being a Patient

The phase of being a patient may be started with the primary diagnosis. During this phase, the major sources of psychologic stress for the patient are the illness itself, the role as a patient, the medical environment, and the variety of specific examinations and therapies.

The intensity of psychologic stress caused by illness is dependent on what recognition and evaluation to the severity and prognosis of illness the patient should give. The entity, characteristics, and severity of illness may affect the recognition and evaluation. On the other hand, the individuality of the patient, i.e., the characteristics of his personality and past knowledge and experience of this kind of illness may affect the recognition and evaluation.

7.1.2.2.3 Phase of Recovery or Rehabilitation

Recovery is when the disease is nearing a cure. If the disease is incurable, the chronic course of disease or abnormal bodily functions will appear. This course is called rehabilitation. Incurable illness, sufferings from uncontrolled symptoms, limitation of normal bodily functions, and psychologic conflict or defeat are the sources of stress for patients in the phase of rehabilitation. The psychologic stress might be so violent that the patients in the phase of rehabilitation are regarded as "disabled in psychologic society." Cancer as a source of stress may produce severe and complex psychologic reaction, because, once a diagnosis of cancer has been established, the patient may live in constant fear that the disease will recur, all measures of therapy may fail, and the disease will run to the terminal stage – death.

7.1.3 Psychologic Components in Patients with Gynecologic Cancers

The basic characteristic of patients with gynecologic cancers is that they are females suffering from cancer. These patients often have special social, emotional, physical, and economic problems. The magnitude of the problems depends on the emotional and psychologic stability of the individual patient. Other facts that may contribute to the extent of the problems depend on how much the patient knows about her condition, her previous experiences with cancer in friends or family, and her family responsibility.

General psychophysiologic components may include the following:

7.1.3.1 Avoidance and Self-defense

7.1.3.1.1 Avoidance

When a person encounters a source of stress and if the course of action the person pursues is to stay well away from the stress source, it is called avoidance. This avoidance often indicates her awareness that something is wrong and that she does not want it confirmed. On the other hand, it may indicate that she is attempting to integrate and handle the threat presented by the symptoms in her own way before being able to cope with such confirmation. Sometimes, the perception of the disease is so frightening that she cannot accept it and reacts as though nothing is wrong. Although it is a subconscious rejection of the threatening situation, her psychophysiologic balance and the relationship between herself and her family can be temporarily maintained.

7.1.3.1.2 Self-defense

When a person is confronted with stress, she sometimes unconsciously ignores or denies it with an attitude of distorting fact or deceiving herself. This psychologic capacity to defend oneself is based on the mechanism of self-defense, which may not only represent a psychologic response but may also control the degree of psychologic stress. Self-defense is composed of the following:

1 Self-defense may severely distort reality in ways of denial, projection, and isolation.
2. Self-defense may moderately distort reality in the modes of transformation, transference, retrogression, and decoration.
3. Self-defense may mildly distort reality in patterns of sublimation, complement, and humor.

In most instances, when a patient knows the diagnosis of cancer, she cannot acknowledge the fact of cancer at a conscious level. Not only does the patient want to define whether she is really suffering from cancer, but she also dreams of having cancer in the early stage, which may be cured radically. Now, let us give an example:

A pelvic mass was found in a 44-year-old gynecologist during her healthy screening examination. When she was aware of the diagnosis of a malignant neoplasm from the doctor's facial expression, she immediately jumped off the examination bed and absolutely denied the diagnosis of a malignant neoplasm with confidence and said: " I am certainly unable to suffer from cancer! The mass palpated is definitely not a malignancy!" Being a gynecologist, her behavior obviously deviates from normal in a negative direction. However, her behavior is in accordance with a normal psychologic self-defense response.

7.1.3.2 Anxiety Reactions and the Extreme Sense of Isolation

Anxiety reactions are probably the most common of all emotional reactions. They often represent a person's nervousness and feelings toward fairly specific crises, and are characterized by fear, worry, and nervousness.

Having passed through the psychophysiologic stage of self-defense, the patient was consciously aware of the reality that she was suffering from cancer.

Awareness of self is heightened as the patient, in essence, surrenders herself for acceptance of therapy and admission to the hospital, when the extreme sense of isolation experienced by the majority of cancer patients would appear. The psychologic withdrawal of others from her immediate environment results in a unique isolation for that patient. She suddenly feels lonely and often feels isolated from her friends, from her husband, and from her family. She is no longer engaged in fulfilling her ambitions. Living longer has no meaning for her. "Dying and death" is waiting for her. She indulges in fantasy. . . . She becomes isolated from the social world. More commonly, she sits alone with a blank expression and does not speak. She looks as if she is compelled to think about her illness. The intensity of the patient's anxiety reactions is dependent on individual characteristics, established patterns of behavior in reaction to stress, family relationships, and what the patient knows about cancer. The entity of the anxiety reaction and the extreme sense of isolation also lead the patient to deny the fact that she has cancer, and she is unable to calm herself in the face of this unexpected fact (of course, it is impossible to calm herself). On the other hand, it is essential that the patient should make a psychologic adjustment and be able to deal with the source of stress.

7.1.3.3 Emotional Release

Anxiety is an internal, subjective experience which is not usually discovered by others. When a person has already recognized the severity of stress and is unable to deal with it, the anxious feeling may turn into an extreme emotional release which is also called an outbreak. The emotional release or outbreak is the important signal for clinical diagnosis of "stress reaction." Having experienced pain from anxiety and solitude, the patient must face the stimulation of illness, the patient's role, the medical environment, and special examination and therapy. All of the sources of stress may cause the emotional conflict in the patient, creating emotional release or emotional outbreak.

The following are the three kinds of basic conflict.

7.1.3.3.1 Approach-Approach Conflict

This conflict is caused by the contradiction between the person's desire and objective condition. A person is attracted by two goals and is anxious to achieve both. However, because of the limitation of the external environment or society, she is forced to select one of these goals. Then, she is in an approach-approach conflict. The more indecisive and the more concerned with the two targets the person is, the more serious the conflict is.

For example, a young female patient suffering from early-stage, low-malignant degree of ovarian cancer desires not only to keep her reproductive function but is also anxious to have the opportunity to eradicate her disease. It is obvious that she is unable to do both, so she is in an approach-approach conflict.

7.1.3.3.2 Avoidance-Avoidance Conflict

In this condition, the person is facing two unacceptable things. If she is planning to avoid one, the other will be unavoidable. It seems that she is in front of a cliff and is being pursued by soldiers.

For example, a patient is suffering from advanced vulva cancer. If the cancer is extensively invading the anus and lower end of the rectum, the decision as to which modality of therapy should be accepted may cause psychologic problems. If vulvectomy and abdominoperineal resection are accepted, she would have to suffer the attack caused by this radical surgery and the problems of post-operative care of an artificial anus. In addition she is also in constant fear of a recurrence of cancer. If she receives radiation therapy, she worries about the effectiveness of radiation on such extensive and invasive disease and she might encounter side effects after the therapy. At this time, she is in avoidance-avoidance conflict.

7.1.3.3.3 Approach-Avoidance Conflict

When a person pursues a goal with a contradictory attitude – both expectancy and refusal – she is in approach – avoidance conflict. The following case history illustrates this condition.

Meng, a 30-year-old nurse, married 2 years ago, was diagnosed as suffering from ovarian cancer, and was referred to surgical intervention. Unfortunately, her husband was studying in the United States. She was so impatient that she wanted to see him at once. However, she was immediately conscious that she should not interfere with his study. Therefore, her willingness to recall her husband produced an approach-avoidance conflict and more severe emotional responses – anxiety, melancholy, and distress.

The above psychologic conflicts inevitably lead to a release of emotion. Some patients are very excited, easily become angry, and are apt to criticize and attack other persons unreasonably. She is often furious with her husband and children and makes various complaints. Sometimes, she is agitated and unwilling to cooperate with the physicians and nurses. Other patients are depressive, disappointed, pessimistic, anxious, and dispirited. She might even commit suicide.

7.1.3.4 Learned Helplessness, Disorders of Cognition, and Decline of Self-Worth

7.1.3.4.1 Learned Helplessness

Learned Helplessness is a complex of learned behavior and an attitude characterized by weakness, incompetence, passiveness, not being able to see an alternative, being at a loss as to what to do, and being in a state of inertia. It will occur if all measures have failed to attack the challenge of sources of stress when the person considers that she does not have the ability to change her present condition.

7.1.3.4.2 Cognition Disorders

Disorders of cognition may be mainly caused by sources of stress in two different ways. Sources of stress may cause psychologic imbalance and harmful emotional responses. On the other hand, sources of stress may directly affect the process of recognized activity. If a person is afflicted with more intensive stress, she will have disorders of cognition in varying degrees. Ye, a 56-year-old professor and head of a department of pediatrics, was diagnosed as having endometrial carcinoma, stage III. She underwent an operation in combination with pre-operative intracavitary radiation, postoperative external radiation, and hormone therapy. Two months later, after her discharge from hospital, metastatic foci to the lung were ascertained by X-ray examination. She considered the foci in the lung as an inflammatory change and asked to be treated with antibiotics. She felt well after the antibiotic therapy. However, she died from pulmonary metastases after a short period. It is obvious that this pediatrician with endometrial carcinoma had cognition disorder.

7.1.3.4.3 Decline of self-worth

Decline of self-worth may directly affect a person's motive to manage the sources of stress, losing confidence and courage to make progress. It has been concluded that working efficiency would be reduced in a person with reduced self-worth, especially those whose self-worth was originally lower than that of normal persons.

The patient with recurrent, metastatic, or terminal cancer already overwhelmed by her own problems appears pessimistic and disappointed, and feels she can no longer carry on normal activities. She may have guilty feelings and blame and the disease on herself because of some forbidden activity. She frequently considers that she has become a burden to her family and her life is no longer meaningful.

7.1.3.5 Disappointed Depressed Phase

When all modalities of treatment have failed to control the cancer, the patient may consider herself as a person in the terminal stage of the disease. Everything being irredeemable, she has been in a state of utter exhaustion and is forced to continue to death. Although the patient is in a state of advanced cancer, hope is also the philosophical ingredient that provides strength for the oft-prolonged period of uncertainty for the patient. For as long as the patient believes she has some degree of control over what is happening to and within her body, the concept of hope is very strong factor in her ability to face whatever the next day holds for her.

7.2 Medical Intervention and Nursing Care of Patients with Gynecologic Cancers

Once a diagnosis of cancer has been established, the patient must not only be treated with biomedical modalities such as surgery, radiation, chemotherapy, and hormonal therapy but also psychophysiologic and social care.

7.2.1 Psychophysiologic Care

7.2.1.1 General Implications for Medical Staff

The medical staff must recognize that there is no blueprint to be followed in dealing with the psychologic problems involved in the course of medical care for patients with cancer. Each patient is unique and must be regarded as one reacting to her disease with feelings, attitudes, concerns, and fears specifically her own.

A warm, interested concern from the medical staff is most important for all patients. It should be rememberd that patients value a smile, friendship, and warmth, since they are needed as much as, and sometimes more than, technical skills. If the patient can receive all the skill, understanding, support, and empathy from the time of admission through her therapy and after discharge, it will facilitate a more rapid rehabilitation for her.

7.2.1.1.1 Sitting Down Beside the Patient

Sitting down means that the physician or nurse allocates sufficient time to listen to the patient's complaints and talk with her. Talking between the medical staff and patient in a friendly way might be a great comfort to the patient, while talking between the medical staff standing in front of the patient and a patient lying on her bed might create an unpleasant atmosphere for the patient because of the hurried attitude and commanding position of the medical staff. The medical staff must remember that any hint that help is grudgingly given will be recognized by the patient, who in turn will deem it worthless.

7.2.1.1.2 Listening to Her

Often the patient desperately wants someone to talk with and listen to her. The epitome of good medical staff is a willingness to listen to them with sympathy and encouragement. Sensitive and understanding medical staff are also willing to spend time teaching the patient and her family and have an insight into the problems, anxieties, and fears of the patient suffering from cancer.

The patient with advanced disease often becomes severely depressed and feels too weak and too tired to get up and talk. While the patient is still in bed, shaking her hands or gently stroking her shoulder or back is a silent conversation which may be helpful to her.

7.2.1.1.3 Paying Attention to Emotional Changes in Patients

It is essential to have enough conversation between the medical staff and patient. Enough conversation depends on the patient's ability to adapt herself to the situation of being a patient with cancer and which examination methods and treatment modalities are given to her. The medical staff who are knowledgeable and who have adequate understanding and empathy for "what the person is going through" will be good at finding out her troubles from her manner of speech, tone of voice, and facial expression and can provide much assistance in her fight against cancer.

7.2.1.1.4 Employing an Attitude of Understanding

The medical staff's awareness that the patient with cancer is subject to recurrences, complications, altered anatomy and physiology, emotional upsets, and prejudices to others will determine the attitude in medical care.

Many patients worry about the loss of money and possible loss of their familiar job or speciality because of their lengthy illness. Others fear death, pain, multilation, rejection by family and friends, and dependency on others. Faced with such devastative threats, the patient may be overwhelmed to the point that she is unable to make sound decisions. She may experience a deep sense of helplessness and seriously contemplate the idea of suicide.

Understanding the patient is of the utmost importance – what she knows, what she does not know, and what she really wants to hear. Knowing her as a person and not a "case" is essential. This means having respect for the dignity of a human being, eliciting her likes and dislikes, and determining what her hopes and plans were before her illness and what her fears and worries are now.

The physician and nurse face a much more difficult and frustrating situation when death is imminent. For the most part, physician and nurse do not know what to say or how to handle the situation when a patient asks: "Doctor, am I going to die?" The answer, of course, is that there is no standard reply. If the medical staff are sure of her feelings and philosophy, the exact words used do not matter, while manner, voice, facial expression, and genuine empathy for the patient are all that matter. However, it is of importance that the physician and nurse observe and evaluate just what her goal is in saying such discouraging remarks. The patient may truly feel that she is in the terminal stage of cancer. For some patients, death is welcome and their expression and willingness also need to be understood.

Death that faces everybody born into this world is unavoidable. Many fear death and many are afraid of talking about death. This has been a fear since ancient times; it has its roots in our very existence. The dying patient and medical staff should be companions in their journey to death. It is just "Death awaiting us all" which is the basis of communication between the dying patient and medical staff and which is the essence of terminal care.

7.2.1.2 How to Explain the Condition of Illness

If the diagnosis of cancer is confirmed, whether or not the patient should be told that she has cancer is still debatable. The consensus is that this is a matter to be decided between the physician, patient, and family, because many people are still unable to deal openly with cancer. In China, the protective medical regimen should be followed, that is the actual situation of illness should be explained to members of the patient's family instead of the patient herself. In the United States, it is a rule that once a diagnosis is ascertained the condition should be told to the patient as soon as possible. It has been agreed that the primary purpose of telling an individual that she has cancer is to create a state of mind which enables the patient to cooperate fully with a minimum of anxiety during therapy and to resume function with a modicum of comfort (Bard 1960).

In Japan another method is advocated. The patient is allowed to understand her condition of illness step by step and eventually accept the reality.

Cancer tends to be a prolonged battle and it may have acute crises and successive but sometimes temporary remissions. When the physician is going to explain what has happened to the patient herself, the best way is to say "It seems that we should have enough preparation to devote ourselves to an enduring battle." This explanation may include the following:

1. The phrase "an enduring battle" does away with the negative "death and dying" attitude. Some patients, after hearing the diagnosis confirmed or after the operation, do fear death, and are rather disturbed.
2. The word "enduring battle" expresses that the patient must go through a tortuous road in the future, since cancer may recur or a new primary lesion may be discovered even after many symptomless years. All of the anti-neoplastic measures will be given to the patients with this kind of long-term illness, especially to those with advanced or recurrent disease. Patients will suffer from physical and psychophysiologic attacks in the course of therapy. Once the patient is well prepared, she will be able to endure the sufferings with a minimum of anxiety.
3. "It seems an enduring battle" expresses that the medical staff will take part in this battle against cancer together with the patients. If "Let us attack cancer

together" is added, the patient might be encouraged who believes that the hope of a speedy recovery is in sight even when she suffers setbacks in the course of therapy.

7.2.1.3 Being Under the Protection of Modern Medicine

When the cancer is recurrent or advanced and all measures have failed including surgery, irradiation, and chemotherapy, the patient may be considered to be in the terminal stage of disease. The medical staff can do nothing more than keep the patient as comfortable as possible until death ensues. The medical staff must try their best to relieve all of the disturbing symptoms such as pain, constipation, vomit and dyspnea in order to encourage the patient to off load her fears about dying and make her believe that she has been protected under modern medicine.

7.2.1.4 Believing in Hope and Taking Part in the Fight Against Cancer

Maintaining conditions of the patients as near normal as possible will undoubtedly help retain their morale. Allowing the patient to do everything she is capable of doing for herself and for her therapy will avert complete loss of hope and increase her dependence on the medical staff.

Hope is the philosophical ingredient that provides strength for the oft-prolonged period of uncertainty for the patient with advanced cancer. The medical staff play a major role in maintaining this ideology. Belief in hope of the patient is often based on awareness by the staff of improved modalities of therapy, increasing curative rate of some neoplastic disorders, and the prolonged survival rate of patients under their care. The empathic flow of hope from the staff is readily detected by the patients. This is especially true when they believe themselves to be an integral part of the health team in fighting against the disease (Buehler 1975).

7.2.2 Physical Care

As soon as endometrial carcinoma has been detected, an appropriate treatment schedule, either radical or palliative therapy, should be drawn up according to the severity of disease. For the incurable patient, the person who cannot be cured with aggressive therapy, palliative and meticulous care should be the vocation of medical staff. For the dying patient, proper care should not be ended. Skilled nursing, relief of pain and distressing symptoms, supportive family counseling, and bereavement care all help permit death with dignity and relative comfort. (Refer also to Chap. 4.)

7.2.3 Social Care

7.2.3.1 Help from Community Resources

Heavy financial burdens are placed on the family of a patient suffering from cancer. Not only is the cost of treatment expensive but many other complex problems also arise during the course of the patient's illness. Many patients and families need assistance, since lack of help may be a major factor in delaying rehabilitation.

In China, the Labour Unions of factories, offices, schools, etc. provide the financial support or temporary loans for working staff or their relatives. The Ministry of Public Health is responsible for overall planning and coordination and provides technical help and materials to local divisions and units. Local units provide assistance to the patient suffering from cancer and her family in meeting the grave problems and heavy financial burden of this serious illness. Local units provide a variety of services available to everyone. Information about cancer, cancer detection, and facilities for diagnosis may be obtained by visiting the local unit in person.

7.2.3.2 Support from the Family

When patients have problems, their families cannot escape involvement. Some families react by being overly solicitous, whereas others reject the patient and her illness. Both types of reaction may be considered normal, and in either case the medical staff can help by accepting the feelings of the family and supporting those of the patient. Many authorities in the fields of psychiatry and clinical psychology have pointed out that where there has been true love and affection and a close network of family associations, the patient will receive the support needed for full rehabilitation. However, if there have been feelings of ambivalence or outright hostility before the diagnosis and therapy, there will be an out-and-out rejection of the patient, and rehabilitation will be greatly hampered. Alert, understanding, and knowledgeable medical staff can frequently elicit these fears and help the family adjust to the difficult situation so that the patient is supported in the course of her therapy.

7.2.3.3 Establishing Community Hospice

A hospice provides a program of palliative and supportive care which recognizes the physical, psychologic, social, and spiritual needs of dying persons and their families. Palliative care is that which provides the most modern and sophisticated treatment to relieve the symptoms and distress of the disease process. The major elements of hospice care for the dying are the following:

1. Symptom control: a thorough but noninvasive assessment, individually titrated drugs regularly administered to control pain and retain alertness, and constant attention to sources and therapies for any discomfort
2. Treating patient and family as a unit of care
3. Available home and inpatient care, 24 h/day, 7 days/week
4. Physician-directed medical services, nurse-directed nursing care, and inter-disciplinary attention to the patient's physical, psychologic, spiritual, and social suffering
5. Volunteers to help the family maintain a normal daily life
6. Continuing bereavement care for the family and support throughout mourning (Blues 1984)

7.3 Euthanasia

7.3.1 Basic Concepts

The medical profession is confronted daily with such legal and ethical dilemmas. Is the physician who practised euthanasia by discontinuing treatment or by administering a lethal drug to a dying patient subjecting her- or himself to civil and criminal liability? Does the patient have a legal right to decide when treatment should be withheld? Who has the legal right to decide the fate of the minor or incompetent terminally ill patient? These questions lead logically to a discussion of euthanasia. The term "euthanasia," taken from the Greek, means literally "good death." In this sense, it might be perfectly acceptable to use the word to describe both allowing the patient to die and mercifully killing her, i.e., active or positive and passive or negative euthanasia.

Active or positive euthanasia is defined as taking positive action to end the life of a terminally ill patient. The physician does something to bring about the patient's death, e.g., the physician gives a cancer patient a lethal injection, which causes the patient's death. Passive or negative euthanasia is the failure to take positive action to prolong the life of an incurable patient. The physician does nothing and allows the patient to die of whatever illness she already has. Active or positive euthanasia helps the patient to die, but the passive or negative form of euthanasia merely "lets the patient go" simply by withholding life-preserving treatment. Euthanasia has been a long-term debatable focus from the medical and ethical view point, even if there have been very few convictions for euthanasia. (Zhang 1988)

Approximately 2500 years ago, Buddhism founded by Sakyamuni advocated Nirvana, which originates from Sanskrit and means oblivion to diseases, troubles, and sufferings. "Pass away in a sitting posture" is the terminal stage of Nirvana, which means that many eminent monks in Buddhism take a bath, change their long gown, and sit in meditation putting their palms together in their terminal period of life. At this stage, their bodies should be under the control of a thought, attaining a lofty realm of oblivion to themselves and leading away from life – a serene voyage to death. (Zhu 1985) Leading away from life achieved by Nirvana might be a happy, gentle, and comfortable death. The aim of Nirvana is so similar to euthanasia that some theologians consider Nirvana as the pioneer of euthanasia.

7.3.2 Quality of Life, Human Suffering, and Euthanasia

Traditional ethics is based upon the conviction of the sanctity of life, which was the classical doctrine of medical idealism in its prescientific phase. The basic elements of the sanctity-of-life ethics are essential for ethical living and cannot be set aside without weakening man's respect for man. They are neglectful of the quality of human life, however.

Biomedical progress is forcing everybody to make fundamental conceptual changes as well as scientific and medical changes. Not only are the conditions of life and death changing, but also definition of life and death have to change to keep pace with the new realities (Fletcher 1973). Life is not an end in itself, independent of other values, and life is worth preserving only if its quality remains intact. Therefore, quality-of-life ethics which advocates the importance of the quality of human life and is in opposition to traditional ethics has emerged as the times required.

Yet the value of human life has not been accurately and quantitatively evaluated. It may only be estimated by the mathematical model. The value of human life is directly proportional to contributions, quality of life, cure rate, and expectancy of life, but inversely proportional to cost.

Value of human life

$$\propto \frac{\text{contributions} \times \text{quality of human life} \times \text{cure rate} \times \text{expectancy of life}}{\text{cost}}$$

It is obvious that being a human is more "valuable" than being alive. A patient in irreversible coma resulting from damage to vital brain centers or in a terminal stage of cancer, whose medical treatment merely prevents the complete cessation of life, without being able to restore independent function of the most basic vital processes, is in such a situation that he or she is no longer a human being, no longer a person, and no longer really alive. (Zhang 1988)

Without a doubt, the only proper care of a patient is to treat him or her as a person, a whole person, and not just as a specimen of biologic life. A fundamental principle of medical ethics is that people be treated with respect; violation of the human person, thus, is unethical. "Letting the helpless patient go" is the code of quality-of-life ethics.

Obviously, the code of quality-of-life ethics is to attack the principle of sanctity-of-life ethics violently. From the principle of sanctity-of-life ethics, the basic task of the physician is to heal and preserve life, to restore health to the sick, to alleviate suffering resulting from disease, excluding any sanction to end the life, or hasten the death, of his patient, as implied in the accepted meaning of euthanasia. The obligation of the physician in a hundred hospitals across the land is from prolonging genuinely human life to only prolonging subhuman dying. Prolonged life by itself is apt to turn into a burden, a change aggravated even more by additional painful sickness. The patient may welcome death either out of exhausion or out of compliance, having reached the stage where she wished for a quiet "beautiful death".

It is better to help the helpless patients escape from such pointless misery than let them die a slow, ugly, and dehumanized death. This is the humanism or personalism which puts humanness and personal integrity above biologic life and function. Certainly, this would help a terminally ill cancer patient to have an apparently peaceful voyage beyond life's frontiers.

The discussion on euthanasia is continuing. A changing public view of this problem may eventually also influence the legal approach. In an attempt to clarify a patient's right to refuse treatment, several state legislatures in the United States are considering the "living will" concept, which is a signed statement requesting that life be not unduly prolonged. The document helps to alleviate both the relatives' anxiety and guilt and the health professionals' obligation to assume that their patients want every effort made to prolong life. A Living Will is distributed by the Euthanasia Educational Council.

In pertinent part, it reads:

Death is as much a reality as birth, growth, maturity, and old age – it is the only certainty of life. If the time comes when I, ————, can no longer take part in decisions for my own future, let this statement stand as an expression of my wishes, while I am still of sound mind.

If the situation should arise, in which there is no reasonable expectation of my recovery from physical or mental disability, I request that I be allowed to die and not be kept alive by artificial means or "heroic measures." I do not fear death itself as much as the indignities of deterioration, dependence, and hopeless pain. I therefore ask that medication be mercifully administered to me to alleviate suffering even though this may hasten the moment of death (Calahica and Hirsch 1984).

The day will come when people will be able to carry a card, notarized and legally executed, which explains that they do not want to be kept alive beyond the human point, authorizing the ending of their biologic processes by any method of euthanasia which seems appropriate.

References

Aguilera DC, Messick JM (1978) Crisis intervention: theory and methodology, 2nd edn. Mosby, St Louis

Bard M (1960) The psychologic impact of cancer III. Med J 118:155

Blues AG (1984) Hospice philosophy of appropriate care. In: Blues AG, Zerwekh JV (eds) Hospice and palliative nursing care. Grune and Stratton, New York 1–9

Buehler JA (1975) What contributes to hope in the cancer patient? Am J Nurs 75:1353–1356

Calahica LA, Hirsh HL (1984) Active and passive euthanasia: medical and legal considerations. In: Carmi A (ed) Euthanasia. Springer, Berlin Heidelberg New York p. 155

Du ZZ (1987) Health, illness and cultural environment. Med Philos 8 (9):1–3

Fletcher J (1973) Ethics and euthanasia. Am J Nurs 73:674–675

Liu DE (1987) The origin and development of medical psychology. Med Philos 8 (4):36–38

Zhanf XQ (1988) Ethical study on the treatment of patient with irreversible coma or terminally ill cancer. Med Philos 9(1): 38–41

Zhu YY (1985) "Euthanasia" and "Nirvana"–several psychological analyses. Med Philos 6 (6) 48–49